Syphilis As AIDS

Robert Ben Mitchell

BANNED BOOKS
Austin, Texas

Library of Congress Cataloging-in-Publication Data

Mitchell, Robert Ben, 1958–
Syphilis as AIDS / Robert Ben Mitchell.
p. cm.
Includes bibliographical references, index.
ISBN 0934411-35-2 : $8.95
1. AIDS (Disease)—Etiology. 2. Syphilis. I. Title.
RC607.A26M57 1990
616.97'92071—dc20 89–18587
CIP

A BANNED BOOK

Published in the United States of America
By BANNED BOOKS
An Imprint of Edward-William Publishing Company
Number 292, P.O. Box 33280, Austin, Texas 78764

ISBN 0-934411-35-2

I dedicate this book to my mother who telephoned me long distance in 1988, at a point when I was very frustrated from working on the manuscript for this book, to yell at me and convince me to never stop, never look back, and never give up.

Contents

Forewords

1. Harris L. Coulter, Ph.D.
2. Stephen S. Caiazza, M.D.

1.

Many of us were raised on Paul de Kruif's *Microbe Hunters*, which popularized the achievements of physicians in taming and conquering diseases. But today we have books like Robert Ben Mitchell's *Syphilis as Aids*—a new literary genre with an altogether different aim. Instead of glorifying the deeds of physicians and medical scientists, it uses the same information in a different way—to go behind the face of the news and seek out the real story.

Mitchell has done an amazing job of amassing, in readable form, hard-to-find information on the causes, symptoms, and treatment of the acquired immune-deficiency syndrome (AIDS) and its links with syphilis. He has gone through the literature on the causal microbe of syphilis, the *Treponema pallidum*, showing how it lives and propagates, how it infects the human host, and how it is, or is not, affected by the medications commonly used to treat it.

Then he demonstrates in minute detail the symptomatic parallels between syphilis and the new disease we call "acquired immune-deficiency syndrome," showing that they are in reality one and the same.

His symptomatic approach to establishing the parallels between syphilis and AIDS is, in my opinion, particularly valuable. Only in this way will we achieve a true understanding of the relations between these two diseases.

Mitchell's interest in AIDS is motivated by his own life experience. Others have written on such diseases as diabetes, arthritis, heart trouble, cancer. In all cases the tone is less one of admiration for the medical profession than of profound distrust of its aims and achievements.

These writers feel they cannot get true, reliable, accurate, or correct information from the medical profession on the diseases of concern to them. They sense that the interests of physicians have diverged from those of the patient, that the physician's goal in life is not necessarily to assuage the suffering of the patient but something else.

Why do many medical consumers today suffer from this thoroughly modern malaise?

In my view it reflects the bureaucratization and politicalization of medical though in the latter decades of the twentieth century.

The physician in American society is no longer a free agent who contracts with the patient to cure his aches and pains. This simple relationship disappeared with the horse and buggy. Today, when health-related expenditures consume ten percent of the U.S. gross national product, the physician has become part of a bureaucracy. He practices medicine with a continuing awareness of being monitored. He cannot use a therapeutic technique which seems to him effective unless he has prior approval from his superiors in the bureaucracy. Mitchell gives an example of this process in the preface.

This sense of no longer controlling their own fate is a source of intense dissatisfaction to physicians themselves who, in most cases, entered this profession with the aim of helping humanity, not of becoming cogs in an all-pervasive bureaucracy. And it is also baneful for the advancement of medical thought. Progress in medicine comes from the initiative of individuals who are in direct contact with patients. These are the front-line troops who know what is really happening. They are the ones who can discard outworn methods or devise new ones as the situation changes. Once our civilization loses this direct input from the soldiers on the firing line and must accept the worn and stale opinions of the generals in the rear, we will be condemned to lose all our wars on disease.

But this is what is happening in the case of AIDS: the only acceptable opinions are those formulated by the small coterie in the National Institutes of Health headed by an individual, Robert Gallo, whose own career, as Mitchell shows, has been studded by incidents of virtually criminal fraud and larceny. The only acceptable treatment is the one which has the imprimatur of these individuals.

But are their interests identical with those of the AIDS sufferers? Many of them have patents on diagnostic procedures, and stock in companies, which stand or fall with the existing viral theory of AIDS. They are bureaucratically and institutionally inhibited from giving a fair hearing to any other theory of the origins and treatment of AIDS.

They have chosen patents over patients.

Since physicians are abnegating their duties, individuals like Robert Ben Mitchell must take up the slack. This he has done in a remarkable way, and I recommend the following pages to all who are interested in a vital and readable account of the relationship between syphilis and AIDS.

Harris L. Coulter, Ph.D.

2.

Bob Mitchell has done us a great service. He has given us, both historically and factually, an accurate, insightful, and detailed overview of the relationship between AIDS and either undiagnosed syphilis or chronic syphilis. This is an important book and one which any of us concerned about the AIDS crisis certainly ought to have and ought to read.

Anyone who has read my own book, *AIDS: One Doctor's Personal Struggle*, knows precisely how I feel about the cause of AIDS. It is multifactorial, with many pathogens contributing ultimately to disease. But Bob Mitchell, in his text and in the speech I gave in Miami which he has been kind enough to reprint in its entirety, explains this well.

There are several points here:

1) That there exists a connection between AIDS and syphilis can no longer be doubted or argued.

2) AIDS need not be inevitably fatal. If we can diagnose early and eliminate those pathogens that we can (like syphilis and now like mycoplasma Incognita), the patient has an excellent chance for survival. But the key here is *early diagnosis*. Diagnosis before the patient looks sick. Before the patient feels sick. Before the patient *is* sick. It is so much easier to take an

infected, but healthy individual and keep him healthy and normal than to try and cure a person too far gone.

A question that often comes up is, how are we going to convince "them," the establishment, of what we believe regarding the relationship between AIDS and treatable co-factors. After all, there are powerful HIV, pharmaceutical, and, of course, AIDS industries out there fully prepared to commit murder in order to advance their financial benefits.

We do it with numbers and with publicity. That publicity is crucial to the effort is an additional reason Mitchell's book is so important.

As far as the numbers are concerned, my own remain solid and are standing both the test of time and the scrutiny of other investigators. Recently, I have expanded my operation to open up an additional one hundred slots. It will take time, and time is life I know, but we will do it. The numbers will grow and grow and become undeniable. Ultimately, working together, we will convince the establishment that we are right.

Another factor we have going for us is time. That is, the first cases of AIDS—then called GRID—were described in 1979. Now think about it—this is 1990. We are well into our second decade of living with AIDS. What have the Big Boys—the experts, the ones with all the money who control all the money and won't let any of us little boys have any—accomplished for the patient in that excess of a decade? The answer does not even have to be spoken: nothing!

This strengthens our hand. Because it is time to begin asking, "If your HIV model has led to nothing but waste and death over longer than a decade, is it not time to begin seriously exploring alternatives?" I would love to see how the Big Boys would answer that one.

Efforts like Bob Mitchell's contribute greatly to what unfortunately is a process of attrition. We simply have to wear them down. We have to outlast them. This is yet another reason Bob's book deserves to be read carefully.

I feel obliged to add a final word about protocols. Blind adherence to rigid protocols is one of the reasons we have such serious problems as AZT toxicity, morbidity, and mortality. We must be flexible. Things change and we must be prepared for change. In fact, we must anticipate change.

In general, though, not much has changed since I devised my antibiotic regimen on that DC-10 returning for the last time from Germany (given later in this book). Subtle changes, yes. But the principles remain the same.

Bob Mitchell has given us a good book. It should be read by every AIDS-interested individual.

Stephen S. Caiazza, M.D.
New York City

Preface

I shall be telling this with a sigh
Somewhere ages and ages hence:
Two roads diverged in a wood, and I—
I took the one less traveled by,
And that has made all the difference.

"The Road Not Taken," Robert Frost

In late 1987 I became involved in a movement in Miami, Florida that focused on the problem of AIDS. A small group of concerned individuals began to congregate at that time around an obscure, yet fascinating idea. It appeared that AIDS, the mysterious epidemic of both our decade and century, was perhaps not a mystery at all. Bits and pieces of literature were starting to surface that suggested the new disease AIDS was possibly an old and recently forgotten disease called syphilis.

At first we paid passing interest to this idea. The initial scraps and pieces of information we received were by themselves of little more than coincidental importance. However, at the end of 1987, we found a book written by Dr. Harris L. Coulter called *AIDS and Syphilis—The Hidden Link*. Coulter too had seen the information we had, plus much more that we had not. It was enough to convince him that syphilis was the most likely cause of AIDS. The so-called AIDS virus was little more than an opportunistic infection taking advantage of an already destroyed immune system—an immune system destroyed by syphilis. Here for the first time was an overall coherent analysis of the possible relationship between AIDS and syphilis.

For our little group in Miami, Dr. Coulter's book was the beginning of a long and torturous journey. His conclusions were not absolute, yet they were so well documented as to warrant more research on our part. Certainly, if one man could amass so much information, then there must be others working in this area.

Our first thought was to see if anyone else had information about the AIDS/Syphilis connection. We spent weeks looking for anything closely related to the issue, desperately trying to find more authorities on the subject. We hoped scientists both inside and outside the medical establishment would be exploring this possibility. With all the national attention given to AIDS, we assumed a connection as feasible as this would be one of the first areas researched.

To our dismay, this was not the case. Only a handful of articles from both medical and popular-press journals were available on the subject.[1] Each one offered a brief summary of one aspect of the AIDS/syphilis connection, yet none was comprehensive enough to establish the validity of the overall relationship between the two diseases. We were dumbfounded. It appeared that there was no large scale research effort to investigate syphilis and AIDS. Everything was geared towards viral theories of AIDS, and therapies based upon viral theories. Without even one major national or international study to eliminate the possibility that syphilis was the real cause of AIDS, all the major medical institutions and research establishments had set their sights on viruses, and viruses only.

Fortunately not all individuals had set their sights so narrowly. Within the scant pieces of literature that existed on the subject, we learned of people like Dr. Klaus Dierig and Dr. Urban Waldthaler in Germany, Joan McKenna in California, and Dr. Stephen Caiazza and Salvatore Catapano in New York City. They too had found enough reason to believe there was more to these two diseases than most people realized. In fact, there was enough data out there to suggest that they were actually one and the same. Yet, while the literature did establish an important relationship between the two, the scientific/medical studies did not, and still do not, publicly exist that prove them to be synonymous with one another. The suggestion was strong, but unproven.

We contacted these researchers, whose names we gleaned from our literary search. We mostly sent letters of encouragement to tell them we believed in what they were doing, even if it was contradictory to the established point of view. To our surprise, we received replies from many of those we wrote. They told us that it was just as important to know whether their ideas were right, as not. They wanted either to establish this possible link as reality, and thus begin solving the AIDS dilemma, or eliminate it before moving on to other ideas. Given the objections and lack of support they received from their professional communities, we considered them very brave.

Our correspondence became quite strong with Dr. Caiazza in particular. We had read some articles about him and were particularly fascinated by his reasoning, research, and results. This correspondence led to his visiting Miami twice in the first quarter of 1988. He met with us and over two hundred other interested individuals to discuss what he was doing. Within a month of his second visit, a dozen physicians between Miami and Fort Lauderdale were using or preparing to use an antibiotic therapy he developed for treating AIDS patients. These physicians realized his work was legitimate enough to justify their trying it. Perhaps in time, enough physicians would get involved that a national effort would result which could determine what AIDS/syphilis connection really existed.

Within two months, all the physicians treating AIDS patients on the antibiotic protocol had stopped using it. Their reasons for stopping were evasive, and none of them said the therapy was hurting the patients. We soon realized that the question was not whether the therapy helped the patients, as they all believed in it enough to start using it in the first place. The question was whether the physicians would lose their licenses to practice medicine if they continued to use this syphilis-based therapy. The drugs being prescribed were common antibiotics that are well known by the medical profession for use against syphilis. Yet, by using these drugs, the doctors were not following guidelines for the treatment of AIDS based upon viral theories. As political and financial concerns received top priority, the physicians, one by one, stopped treating their patients with antibiotics.

It was apparent that no matter how persuasive the argument for a possible AIDS/syphilis connection, investigation into this link would not be allowed at the expense of viral research. Despite all the conflicting evidence, some supporting and some denying a viral cause of AIDS, the viral theorists had a firm grasp of the minds and money invested in AIDS. No other point of view would be allowed any significant portion of either. To us this was bad science. We could not understand why a well-known factor like syphilis was not thoroughly researched before the medical profession put all their eggs into the viral basket.

Not only was the medical establishment convinced that AIDS was caused by a virus, but we also realized that most lay people believed this too. As the local doctors lost interest, so did most other local people, including the AIDS patients. People were willing to accept whatever they were told, and if one day they were told syphilis and the next day they were told virus, so be it. Today, viral thinking is the vogue, and syphilis has been forgotten again.

The acceptance of the AIDS virus has gotten to the point that most people cannot separate the disease from this theorized causative agent. Even with all the evidence that disputes the HIV virus as the basis for the disease, people assume that proof exists that it causes AIDS. People assume that if you have AIDS you must also have the AIDS virus. People assume that if you have the AIDS virus you will die of AIDS.

With all the frustration our group faced in Miami, we still could not accept the viral theories, as our literary research provided no proof-positive it was true. On the other hand, we compiled a staggering amount of data that supported the syphilis theory, and continued to be amazed that no national or international effort was aimed at either proving or disproving it. After all, no one was saying it was true; we were simply stating, and continue to state, that there's enough information currently available to justify large scale attention to the link between syphilis and AIDS.

A few weeks after the doctors stopped using the antibiotic protocol for treating their AIDS patients, our group slowly disbanded. Most of us were emotionally and/or financially drained from our experience. We were disappointed that our hard work had not received the attention we felt it deserved. However, from the beginning, we had set two goals.

Our first goal was to determine if there was enough current scientific and medical literature to support the theory about syphilis and AIDS. The second goal was to share this literature with others, if it did exist. We hoped our sharing would inspire continued research into the connection, research by the kinds of minds and institutions that could prove or disprove our contention once and for all.

We did find an overwhelming amount of literature that supported the link between syphilis and AIDS, and we did share it with others. In this sense we knew we had successfully completed our goals. Unfortunately, people we shared our information with chose to ignore it, and no new research resulted from our efforts. In this respect, our success was ultimately a failure.

During the subsequent months, I spent time contemplating why our efforts had not caused others to get involved. I realized that our defeat was not from lack of trying. There was obviously some very good reason why nothing other than viral research would be accepted within the spectrum of AIDS. The question was what or who could possibly gain from ignoring the syphilis connection. There were many lives lost and still at stake in this issue, with projections that the disease has the potential to halt worldwide population growth by the end of the century, less than two decades away. Something extremely important must be involved to tunnel-vision AIDS research so narrowly.

In my search for answers, I began to realize that the experimentation done with AIDS patients might not be designed for their benefit. Though it is their lives that are in immediate threat from this epidemic, their health is likely being sacrificed for areas of interest that have little to do with their pain and suffering. Along with an in-depth look at the intimate relationship between syphilis and AIDS, this book will explore how this relationship is possibly being exploited, and lives being wasted, in a masterpiece of genocidal subterfuge.

References

1. Mike Smith, "The New Syphilis," *The New York Native*, 12/28/87, 16–17.

Acknowledgments

I am very grateful to the staffs of the University of Miami Calder Medical Library, the Miami-Dade Community College Medical Center Campus Library, the Dade County Main Library, and Lambda Passages Bookstore (Miami). Their expertise and help were invaluable in compiling the data upon which this text is based. Also, I wish to thank Bob C. for his tireless pursuit of information, and my lover Omar for his patience and support while I pursued completion of this text.

Introduction

This book has been written in response to an ever increasing international crisis that affects humanity as a whole. As an individual, I have found myself caught up in the issue of AIDS only within the last few years. It has, however, been epidemic as far back as ten years. My late involvement in this problem is perhaps indicative of the fear and lack of interest most people take towards AIDS. Unfortunately, hiding from the problem will not make it go away.

The problem of AIDS is complex and multi-faceted. On the surface, it would appear to be a sexually transmitted disease afflicting specific minorities. This oversimplified analysis suggests the justified foisting of behavioral modification upon these minorities. However, this narrow-minded solution has not, and will not solve the problem of AIDS. More than a disease, AIDS involves many factors beyond general biology, including a wide array of social attitudes, economic influences, and political interests. To ignore any of these parts of the whole, is to miss the broad and complex issue of AIDS. Perhaps, however, it is possible to find a common thread that weaves all of these factors together and binds them into the killer plague of our time. If so, this thread would be ignorance.

More than anything else, ignorance stands in our way of stopping the killer AIDS. Ignorance stands behind most, if not all, of the many factors that have created and continue to nurture the spread of this disease. From the short-sightedness of social attitudes to the corrupting economic pressures of individuals and institutions, ignorance drives AIDS onward like power drives an evil emperor. It is not the consequence of any one man, woman, or child, but the collective ignorance of many people and many societies of people that spreads this disease.

Replacing ignorance with understanding and compassionate action is certainly the first step towards a world without AIDS.

Unfortunately, man has proven to be an animal that lives and dies by ignorance. History has recorded this over and over again, in barbaric and inhumane events throughout our evolution. Today we stand at an important turning point in that evolution. We have the opportunity to work towards a mutual solution to AIDS, or we can continue to ignorantly use it as a weapon against one another. Our collective response to this dilemma will determine the path we take. Just maybe, we can do something different this time and all be better for having made the effort.

Chapter 1

Overview

I am afraid that the medical establishment has totally locked into the HIV theory of AIDS. To back away from it now would be to compromise themselves in the eyes of the public, would mean that hundreds of millions of dollars in research funds had been misallocated, etc. So they will fight against the syphilis theory until the end.

Dr. Harris L. Coulter, in a letter to the author

AIDS has been a medical enigma since the first cases started to appear in the late 1970s. In its brief history to date, it has proven to be one of the deadliest foes ever known to mankind. Compared to other causes of death, it has yet to attain the fatality of cigarette smoking which claims approximately 1000 Americans daily. However, by August 1988 there had already been over 40,000 known deaths[1] from the disease, and the numbers have continued to rise at an alarming rate.

The term "known deaths" is an important one. It stems from the fact that the American CDC (Center for Disease Control) will never receive reports on all deaths caused by this or any other disease. The CDC relies on the street-level physician to report AIDS related deaths to its headquarters in Atlanta, Georgia. Often, however, these deaths are not reported to the CDC, most often to protect the surviving family members from social or financial hardships.[2] According to Dr. Paula Sparti, a Miami physician with many AIDS patients, "Most community practitioners don't report because there's really no guarantee in terms of confidentiality or anti-discrimination . . . They're [AIDS patients] already facing a horrible disease . . . For us to put them in jeopardy of losing their job [*sic*] or the place [*sic*] they're living, it's just not reasonable."[3] For this reason, the CDC uses the term "known deaths" in recognition of the fact that they receive reports on only a percentage of the total number of "all deaths" caused by a disease. Therefore, the actual deaths from AIDS is likely far in excess of the number reported.

In addition to the number of people already dead from AIDS, it is predicted that we have seen only the tip of the iceberg, in terms of its ferociously lethal appetite. John Platt, a biophysicist who has taught at the University of Chicago, MIT, Harvard and the University of Paris, made the following estimates in an article published by *The Futurist* magazine in late 1987. By the end of the decade, according to the article, AIDS could kill more American men than have died in all our wars. Its influence may be so drastic that by 1995, the size of the U.S. population may actually be decreasing, with the death toll reaching fifty million worldwide before the year 2000. In ten to twenty years, whole nations, especially poorer third world nations, may be eradicated as world population growth ceases.[4] Truly these are horrifying prospects.

How could such profound devastation be looming upon our horizon when we live in an era of unparalleled enlightenment? We have at our disposal the greatest scholars of medicine and science that have ever lived. With dollars and minds aimed at a microscopic virus, ten years of experiment after experiment have not provided a cure for AIDS, and there is none foreseen as available in time to stop predictions by Platt and others from becoming reality. It may be, however, that it is not a lack of ideas and wealth that stands in our way of preventing this disaster.

Mankind has often proven to be his own worst enemy when in the pursuit of knowledge. Galileo Galilei (1564 –1642) is a prime example of this. He was the first to propose that the planets orbited around the sun at the center of our solar system. Countless astronomical observations by himself and others proved his theory correct. Today, children are taught this fact in early grade school. However, while alive, Galileo was persecuted for his beliefs and theories, for they were not what the ruling establishment of his time wanted to hear. In the 1500s, the church controlled the hearts and minds of mankind, and they believed the sun and planets revolved around man's earth at the center of the solar system. The best scholars were employed to make the facts fit the church's theory, with elaborate mathematical schemes to account for nature's unwillingness to do as man commanded. Unfortunately for Galileo, he chose to make the theory fit the facts, and it would take the church nearly four centuries to admit its error in judgement upon him.

Today, the church's dogma is no longer the leading influence of man's science that it was in the 1500s. Though still significant, it has taken a back seat to an establishment of doctors from medical and other scientific fields. Yet the ability to be wrong on a grandiose scale is no less a fault of the current rulers than it was of those that persecuted Galileo. The thalidomide, swine flu vaccine, and other medical disasters stand as testament to the fallibility of our sciences, and AIDS may prove to be the most lethal of modern medicine's mistakes.

When faced with any problem, rational analysis of known factors has proven to be the best starting point from which to attempt to find a solution. It should not be surprising that rational analysis is at the heart of what is called the scientific method. This method, which guides all scientific investigation, lays down precise rules of observation and experimentation upon which theories are built. The goal of this method is to find answers based upon facts of nature, not man's imagination. If the church had used the scientific method, Galileo's genius would have been recognized in the 1500s.

The investigation of AIDS has been governed by the scientific method. However, a multitude of experimental observations and published results in the medical community show that a fundamental error may have taken place in studying this disease. This error centers on the very cornerstone of AIDS research, that a virus causes AIDS.

It is highly probable that AIDS is not caused by a virus, but by a bacterium called TP (Treponema pallidum—the causative agent of syphilis). This research will lay out the evidence for challenging the current foundation of AIDS research. There is not enough data in this book to definitively state once and for all that TP causes AIDS. The goal of this book, however, is to show that the correlation between the two diseases is so strong that a national and/or international effort must be made to determine the AIDS/syphilis connection exactly. Should TP ultimately prove to be the culprit, inexpensive and curative treatment for AIDS may be available within a few years, and a larger disaster than has already happened, prevented.

References

1. The CDC number of known deaths from AIDS was 40,090 as of August 22, 1988. This figure was obtained from the National AIDS Hotline (1-800-342-2437), which receives monthly updates from the CDC.
2. Allen Chase, *The truth about STD* (William Morrow and Co., Inc.: 1983), 21, 43.
3. "Doctors Fail to Report AIDS, Fearing Discrimination," UPI, Miami, 2/21/88.
4. John Platt, "The Future of AIDS," *The Futurist*, vol. 21, no. 6 (November–December 1987): 10–17.

Chapter 2

The Emperor Has No Clothes

. . . the one who finally dared to tell the truth was a black servant who said to the king, 'My Lord, I am a poor man and have nothing to lose. Therefore I say to you, either I am blind or you are going about naked'. . . But the trumpets went on blaring and the cymbals went on clashing, so what could the emperor do except go marching straight ahead? And the royal chamberlains held up the invisible train as high as if it had been real.

The Emperor's New Clothes[1]

AIDS, the epidemic, has been underway for over a decade. During this time, there has been a dramatic rise in the number of cases, and a corresponding rise in the interest researchers have taken in understanding the disease. Unfortunately, given the years, knowledge, and financing available to modern medicine, no cure has been discovered, nor is one predicted to be found anytime in the near future. Yet, there is a force which drives research forward: HIV. It commands the thoughts and resources of this nation, and many others, but produces few results. It may be, therefore, a naked emperor, with little substance upon which to base such control.

The illnesses and deaths from AIDS, which most people would like to stop, are the terrible effects caused by this disease. Yet, in order to stop these effects, the cause itself must first be found. Most everyone today is in agreement that HIV is the causative agent of AIDS, although, as the premise for the disease's origin, it has done little to provide scientists with the essential insights needed to stop AIDS. The man often given undue credit for discovering the virus in late 1983, Dr. Robert Gallo of the NCI (National Cancer Institute), speculated at the 88th annual meeting of the American Society for Microbiology that a herpes virus co-factor may be required to help HIV cause AIDS.[2] For years Gallo has proclaimed that HIV was the one and only cause of the disease and, his words, like theologic dogma of the middle ages, have been accepted without question. Now, five years from his claiming rights to the HIV discovery, Gallo himself is no longer sure of HIV's true role in AIDS.

Though he has done much credited and noteworthy work in other areas, as a mentor for today's AIDS researchers, Gallo's influence has been undeserved, and possibly tragic. Historically, his zealous attitude and overbearing manner have left him with a history of unreliable research. In 1976, before the AIDS crisis, he stated he had discovered a new virus. However, the scientific results upon which this claim was based were actually due to contamination of his experiments, and not a new virus.[3] False statements like this are detrimental to the advancement of understanding diseases. The alleged origins of the HIV virus suffer this same problem. In February of 1988, Bob Stein, a science writer for United Press International, reported that researchers at the New England Primate Research Center had determined that the theory claiming HIV to have originated in green monkeys of Africa was based upon experiments contaminated by extraneous viruses from Rhesus macaque monkeys. According to the article, because of this revelation of error, "the leading theory of the origin of the AIDS virus was thrown into doubt . . . it is now totally up in the air again where the virus originated . . ."[4]

In addition to Gallo's history of faulty research methods, there is substantial evidence which shows that HIV was not discovered by him, but by a team of scientists under the direction of Dr. Luc Montagnier in France. The French called their isolate of the virus LAV, while Gallo named it HTLV-III, both being names for the same virus, just as "humanity" and "mankind" refer to the same thing. Shortly after being coined, the terms LAV and HTLV-III were replaced by the name commonly used today: HIV. In his book *The Band Played On*, Randy Shilts gives a detailed account of how Dr. Gallo was to receive credit for the labor of the French.[5] In summary of Shilts, it seems the French had not only discovered the virus a year before Gallo's claim, but they actually sent him samples of LAV shortly after isolating it. The implications of Gallo's scientific plagiarism were revealed by Montagnier during a 1985 AIDS conference in New York City. Gallo even went so far as to use electron microscope photographs of French LAV, claiming them to be pictures of his HTLV-III.[6] How a man with a history of research errors, thievery, and contradictory statements became the modern guru of AIDS is in itself a miracle of modern medicine.

Another fascinating paradox in the HIV story is the original motivation which led researchers to narrow their search for the cause of AIDS to just viruses. In the early days of 1980, viruses were among a number of germ suspects for science to investigate. According to Shilts, the elimination of non-viral organisms, including syphilis, was begun when hemophiliacs were found to have contracted AIDS from contaminated factor VIII, a blood component essential for proper blood clotting.[7] Agencies like the American Red Cross isolate factor VIII from healthy blood donors to give to people suffering from hemophilia caused by deficiencies in this factor. The filtering process used during the preparation of factor VIII was believed to prevent anything larger than a virus from being passed along to the hemophiliacs. This, however, is not true.

Viruses are extremely small in size. They are measured in microscopic units called nanometers (one meter is equal to one billion nanometers). They range from under 100 nanometers in diameter, to up to 500 nanometers in diameter, depending on the virus. HIV belongs to a class of viruses called retroviruses, which are round and commonly up to 130 nanometers in diameter.[8] On the other hand, Treponema pallidum (TP), the causative agent of syphilis, is a bacteria whose size is measured in units larger than nanometers, called microns (one meter is equal to one million microns, and one micron is equal to one thousand nanometers). TP is a long, corkscrew shaped organism. Its length is commonly in the range of 10 to 13 microns, however, its diameter can be as small as 0.1 microns, which equals 100 nanometers,[9] smaller than the diameter of a retrovirus. Treponemas are known to be capable of migrating through filters that have pore sizes of 200 nanometers in diameter, as is outlined in *Bergey's Manual of Systemic Bacteriology.*[10] Given that they are highly flexible and mobile organisms, it is this diameter, not the length of the TP, which is so important in determining whether or not a filtering process will remove the syphilis bacteria. As the diameter of TP can be smaller than the diameter of HIV (100 and 130 nanometers respectively), it would appear feasible that any path through which the virus could pass, the bacteria could pass through also. Filtering that would not catch the HIV virus, therefore, would not catch the TP bacterium. The differences between what the filters were believed capable of removing and what they can actually remove are lethal, and leave open the possibility that the hemophiliacs may have received syphilis along with their factor VIII.

Given all the discrepancies between the myths and reality behind the discovery of HIV, it is not surprising to find an NCI-sponsored study which shows why HIV cannot be the cause of AIDS. Professor Peter H. Duesberg works for the Department of Molecular Biology and Virus Laboratory of the University of California in Berkeley. In March of 1987 he published the results of a research grant sponsored by the National Cancer Institute and the National Institutes of Health. His conclusion was, "Indeed the virus [HIV] is not sufficient to cause AIDS." [11] He based his finding upon the following research results:

1) Annually, less than 6% of those infected with HIV go on to develop symptomatic AIDS.
2) The disease AIDS has a latency period of 5 years, but HIV virus attains pathogenic (disease causing potential—not AIDS) and replication maturity within a few days or weeks of its production.
3) There is no gene in HIV that accounts for the ability of the virus to lay dormant inside the human body, yet there is an extremely long latency period between infection with the virus and the onset of AIDS.
4) All other viruses have high titers (concentrations within the body) when they cause disease, but HIV titers are always low, even in carriers with symptomatic AIDS.
5) Viruses, by definition, are cell-free infectious agents. Contamination with viral particles, without body cells, is sufficient to cause disease. It is for this reason that viral diseases are spread by casual contact

methods like sneezing. Contrary to this, AIDS is only transmissible by exchange of human body fluids which contain cells, and not by means of casual contact.

Duesberg has never claimed HIV has nothing to do with AIDS, but merely that the virus is not capable of being the fundamental cause of the disease. If it were the cause of AIDS, then symptoms of the disease should appear shortly after the virus infects the body and is present in large numbers, but this does not happen. Therefore, HIV is most likely just another opportunistic infection taking advantage of an already destroyed immune system. Dr. Gallo's own experiments with HIV support this, as up to early 1988 he had never been able to grow the virus in blood cells of healthy individuals, but only in cells drawn from people already suffering from leukemia, a cancerous affliction of the immune system.[12] In a *Wall Street Journal* article titled "The AIDS Debate That Isn't," journalist Katie Leishman gives a layman's review of Duesberg's reasoning about HIV. She also describes how scientists who believe HIV to be the cause of AIDS have avoided confronting Duesberg and his research results. Though asked to speak before the Presidential Commission on HIV during their 1988 February hearings in New York City, according to Leishman, one of the commissioner's staff reported that Duesberg's invitation to speak was for the purpose of discrediting him. The results of his attendance at the hearings, however, backfired on the commission. In the end, commission member Frank Lilly, chairman of the genetics department of Albert Einstein College of Medicine, admitted "scientists have offered no definitive mechanism by which HIV destroys the immune system and that retroviruses classically do not kill cells [T-cells]." [13] At the time, Dr. Lilly's statement was well known by those in the AIDS administration. With regards to this, in December of 1987, Dr. William Blattner, an NCI epidemiologist, stated, "The mechanism through which Human Immunodeficiency Virus brings about extensive destruction of immunological functions is unknown." [14]

If HIV is not responsible, then what starts AIDS? According to Leishman's article, "Mr. [*sic*] Duesberg allows that syphilis may play a key role in many cases of AIDS." [15]

References

1. Jean Van Leeuwen, *The Emperor's New Clothes*, With text adapted from Hans Christian Andersen and other sources (Random House: 1971).
2. Rosemary Goudreau, "Highly Contagious Herpes Virus Linked to Cancer, AIDS," *The Miami Herald* (5/11/88): 1A.
3. Randy Shilts, *The Band Played On* (St. Martin's Press: 1987), 270.
4. Bob Stein, "Origins of AIDS in Doubt," UPI, 2/17/88, Boston.
5. Shilts, *op. cit.*, 528–531.
6. Mike Salinas, "Kidnapping a Virus," *The New York Native* (3/30/87): 13.
7. Shilts, *op. cit.*, 115–116.
8. Fields, *Virology* (Raven Press: 1985), 237.
9. Mandell, Douglas Jr., and Bennett, *Principles and Practices of Infectious Diseases* (John Wiley and Sons: 1979), 1820.
10. William and Wilkins, *Bergey's Manual of Systemic Bacteriology* (Holt, et. al.: 1984), 1:50.
11. P.H. Duesberg, "Retroviruses as Carcinogens and Pathogens, Expectations and Reality," *Cancer Research*, 47 (3/1/87): 1199–1220.
12. Katie Leishman, "AIDS and Syphilis," *The Atlantic* (January 1988): 21.
13. Katie Leishman, "The AIDS Debate That Isn't," *The Wall Street Journal* (2/26/88): 14.
14. John Laruitsen, "Saying no to HIV," *Christopher Street*, issue 118, vol. 10, no. 10 (December 1987): 34.
15. Leishman, *op. cit.*, *The Wall Street Journal*.

Chapter 3

The Syphilis Theory

I can't think of a single major medical advance that occurred in an atmosphere of double-blind placebo-control studies with the clear support of the medical establishment behind it, . . . Every advance had occurred with someone with some decent thinking behind their work trying something new.

Dr. Kerby Stewartt[1]

The syphilis theory postulates Treponema pallidum (TP), the bacterium responsible for syphilis, as the cause of AIDS. It is based upon the following:

1). Both syphilis and AIDS are transmitted (spread) by the same means.
2). Both syphilis and AIDS follow the same pathogenic pathways, producing the same signs and symptoms of illness.
3). Both syphilis and AIDS are epidemic in the same human populations.
4). Syphilis, historically, has appeared with AIDS-like ferocity prior to the 1900s.
5). The tests used to diagnose syphilis are woefully inaccurate and unreliable.
6). Because of the types and dosages of antibiotics used, the American therapeutic protocol for syphilis is temporary-symptomatic treatment only, not curative.

These ideas are radical for our times. Even with all the inconsistencies of the viral theory, few people are willing to consider anything other than HIV as the cause of AIDS. Yet, given our current crisis, we need new, radical ideas now more than ever. The solutions to AIDS are waiting for us somewhere in the future, with only our ignorance and inflexibility standing in our way of finding them. Those keen to meet the challenge will survive.

While Professor Duesberg, with support from the NCI and NIH, has shown HIV incapable of causing AIDS, it has been the responsibility of other researchers to clarify and demonstrate the role syphilis plays in the disease. Drs. Klaus Dierig and Urban Waldthaler, of Augsberg, Germany, deserve much credit for their initial work in this area. However, this discussion will focus on three Americans: Joan McKenna, Dr. Stephen Caiazza, and Salvatore Catapano.

McKenna, a research physiologist and cofounder of the Institute for Thermobaric Studies in Berkeley, California, became interested in the connection between syphilis and AIDS during the early 1980s. "Unmasking AIDS: Chemical Immunosuppression and Seronegative Syphilis," her research results into the connection, was published in 1986. In it, she focused on the two groups most commonly associated with AIDS: American homosexuals and African Heterosexuals. No other community has been more devastated by AIDS than these two. In addition to their being overwhelmed by AIDS, McKenna established three important similarities between them which support the syphilis theory. The foremost of these links is that both groups were epidemic hot-beds of infectious syphilis before the AIDS crisis, and are still so infected today. McKenna estimates "that more than 60% of the gay community has a history of syphilis and 90% of those with AIDS have had one or more syphilitic infections." [2] An accurate estimate of the comparative infection rate among Africans is difficult to obtain, due to the tense and continually changing political face of the continent. Nevertheless, in her paper, McKenna states the percentage "is considerably higher than in Europe and the USA." [3] It is generally agreed that syphilis and yaws, a disease related to syphilis and caused by a subspecies of TP,[4] are epidemic in Africa, with approximately 80% of the population believed still infected beyond the first half of this century.[5] Though no reference has been found of the current percentage, there is little reason to believe there has been a significant change in this figure, with syphilis, like AIDS, epidemic upon the African continent. Considering that both diseases are spread by the same means and produce the same signs and symptoms in humans, McKenna's finding the two diseases epidemic in both communities provides critical confirmation of the syphilis theory. Had syphilis or AIDS been absent from either of the groups, the connection between the two diseases would have been broken.

McKenna's second link between the gays and Africans is their abuse of antibiotics. These drugs, which in and of themselves can impair normal immune system functions,[6] can be purchased over-the-counter in many third-world nations. Individuals, with little knowledge of their application or side effects, are left to play doctor with one of the most over-used and misunderstood medicines of our time. United States homosexuals, on the other hand, were given countless antibiotic prescriptions for a never ending multitude of varied and often simultaneous reasons, among them syphilis. In addition, gays of the pre-AIDS era showed an intense proclivity for every recreational drug imaginable, with McKenna listing over a dozen of them. The ability of these "fun" drugs to weaken and damage the immune system compounded antibiotic immunosuppression. Unfortunately, the use of antibiotics by both groups provided symptomatic relief only, and did not remove the underlying cause of syphilis: TP. This left the bacterium hidden inside their bodies where it later produced devastating results: AIDS.

The interaction between antibiotics and the immune system was to also play a role in McKenna's third discovery: approximately 33% of the syphilitic subjects studied in both groups were seronegative for syphilis. Put simply, one-third of the syphilis in the gays and Africans could not be detected using standard laboratory blood tests. This misdiagnosis was partially due to chemical immunosuppression. The physical signs and symptoms of syphilis appeared over and over again. However, doctors would not identify TP as the cause due to their over-reliance on these unreliable tests. Thus, an old ailment masqueraded itself as a mysterious new syndrome.

In addition to establishing syphilis, chemical suppression of the immune system, and seronegativity as important factors in AIDS, McKenna helped guide another researcher, Dr. Stephen Caiazza, in his initial investigations into the syphilis-AIDS connection. Caiazza, who received awards for excellence in immunological research during medical school at New York University, has also completed a fellowship in immunology research sponsored by the NIH. He has specialized in AIDS and related disorders since 1982, and in 1985 became interested in the possible role syphilis played in the disease. Shortly after speaking with McKenna, Caiazza went to Germany in the latter part of 1986 to study with Drs. Dierig and Waldthaler. His time overseas provided Caiazza with valuable information and confirmation about his ideas concerning TP. In addition, building on the work of the two German doctors, Caiazza developed a long range treatment protocol for AIDS, based upon new syphilis antibiotic regimens (see appendix A).

Caiazza's work, like that of others who have strayed from the HIV herd, has been harshly criticized by his peers, and he has been continually monitored, to the point of harassment, by the New York State Health Department since his return from Europe in early 1987. He began treating his AIDS patients on the syphilis protocol that year, and the preliminary results of his treatment were published in January of 1988. Titled, "Chronic Spirochetal Infection and the Pathogenesis of AIDS," [7] it was the first presentation of the syphilis theory by a practicing physician in a medical journal. It included impressive results on ten of his sickest patients with full-blown AIDS, stating complete resolution of the PCP, thrush, encephalopathy, colitis, night sweats, and malaise associated with their illness. Also, there were improvements noted in all cases involving adenopathy and weight loss, and two of the three cases of Kaposi's Sarcoma were receding, with the third being stable.

Caiazza notes that even with these significant improvements, this is not definitive proof that antibiotics will cure AIDS. It is, however, a critically important step into areas and ideas we desperately need to investigate. He hopes continued success with his patients will provide the impetus needed for others to begin this kind of research nationwide. In 1988, he was into the second year of trials with the syphilis protocol. During a visit to Miami, he noted that while using antivirals his patients died at a rate of one per week. With his new regimen, he was proud to announce that over the period of a year, he had only lost one[8] (see appendix B).

Dr. Caiazza's success is grounded in his ability to look beyond the surface of our crisis into its fundamental roots. There he has found a viral house of cards, and, like McKenna, has chosen to build his work on a more solid foundation.

Salvatore Catapano, another AIDS researcher, has also found the syphilis theory worthy of investigation. Catapano, a medical researcher with over forty years experience working with venereal diseases and cancer, believes syphilis to be the fundamental cause of AIDS. In a detailed account of his life and work, journalist Katie Leishman describes how he came to this conclusion.[9] A particularly notable part of the article tells about his service in the navy at Princeton University during World War II. Albert Einstein was also at Princeton then, and the two were to spend many hours together enjoying each other's company. At one point, Einstein invited Catapano to his laboratory where the physicist showed him how to mathematically correct for errors in an unreliable urinalysis test being used at the time. It was a friendship that would shape Catapano's thinking and life forever.

During WWII, according to Leishman, Catapano found himself continually confronted with the paradoxes in the diagnosis and treatment of syphilis. Penicillin, believed to be the magic bullet and wonder drug that would eradicate TP, did not always work when used as prescribed. In addition, the tests for syphilis diagnosis did not always give expected results after the penicillin therapy, as many men still showed positive test readings for syphilis infection. Finally, during a brief tour of duty as a laboratory technician on a naval hospital ship in the Pacific, Catapano saw the unusual signs and symptoms of a tropical disease named yaws, which is also caused by the TP bacterium. In the early 1980s he would see these manifestations again, but the disease causing them would be called AIDS.

After the war, due to family members who had died or were dying of cancer during his service in the navy, Catapano changed the focus of his research, determined to find a cure for cancer. Guided by something Einstein told him while at Princeton—"Knowledge is what you remember when you forget what you learned in books." [10]—Catapano decided to forego the drug and radiation therapies then popular in medical texts, in favor of studying the effects immune-system-stimulating vaccines would have on tumors. He was to try multitudes of dosage regimens with a variety of medications before finally being successful with typhoid vaccine. Over a period of several years, upon his request, researchers at the National Cancer Institute confirmed Catapano's typhoid vaccine regimen as both reducing cancer tumors and stimulating immune system production of T lymphocytes (T-cells).

In 1982, the NCI-confirmed abilities of his typhoid vaccine protocol lead Catapano to believe it would help stimulate the damaged immune systems of AIDS patients. Working with a licensed physician and voluntary patients, his results were encouraging, as in many cases a total remission of nearly all signs and symptoms was achieved by controlled vaccine injection. Leishman's article tells how this new application of the typhoid vaccine entitled Catapano to patent his discovery, for which the U.S. patent office granted him patent number 4,711,876, published in December of 1987.[11] It is currently one of only three U.S. patents for the treatment of AIDS, with the other two belonging to Burroughs-Wellcome (AZT) and Sereno Pharmaceutical Partners (thymus extract).

While treating AIDS patients with the vaccine, Catapano became suspicious of what really was causing the disease. He had seen Kaposis sarcoma many years before at the Brooklyn Naval Hospital. Then the patients were elderly European men, the group most likely to be struck by what was then considered a rare sarcoma. The sarcomas of his AIDS patients, however, did not resemble these. They were more like the skin lesions he had seen during his tour of duty in the Pacific, which were caused by the syphilis related disease, yaws. Also, he realized the PCP of AIDS patients resembled the pneumonia of wartime soldiers who were unsuccessfully treated for repeated outbreaks of syphilis. Given the multiple infections and reinfections most AIDS patients had with syphilis and other STD's (e.g. gonorrhea), he was convinced the bacterium, and not the virus, was the primary immunosuppressing factor in AIDS. Added to the highly fallible diagnostic tests still used today for syphilis, and the inability of sub-curative doses of immunosuppressive antibiotics to eradicate TP, Catapano found his research, like McKenna's and Caiazza's, supports the syphilis theory of AIDS.

It is appropriate at this point to include mention and praise of Dr. Harris L. Coulter, author of *AIDS and Syphilis—The*

Hidden Link.[12] As a medical historian, his book was the first to elucidate the connection between these diseases, and has been an immense influence on my understanding of our crisis. It is must reading for anyone interested in this area of research, and includes exclusive at-length interviews with Joan McKenna and Dr. Caiazza. To many, this book has, and will, serve as a guiding light into the future.

References

1. Katie Leishman, "The AIDS Debate That Isn't," *The Wall Street Journal* (2/26/88): 26.
2. Joan McKenna, "Unmasking AIDS: Chemical Immunosuppression and Seronegative Syphilis," *Medical Hypothesis*, vol. 21 (1986): 425.
3. *Ibid*, 424.
4. *Bergey's Manual of Systematic Bacteriology* (Holt, et. al.: 1984), 1:50–51.
5. Paul D. Hoeprich, *Infectious Diseases*, 2nd ed. (Harper and Row Publishers: 1977), 824.
6. Dr. Harris L. Coulter, *AIDS and Syphilis—The Hidden Link* (North Atlantic Books and Wehawken Book Company: 1987), 43–46.
7. Dr. S. Caiazza, "Chronic Spirochetal Infection and the Pathogenesis of AIDS," *Quantum Medicine* (January 1988).
8. Dr. Caiazza visited Miami on March 13, 1988, and gave a presentation of his research results before an audience of approximately two hundred people. The event was covered by all local television network affiliates, and produced immense interest locally in the treatment of AIDS with his syphilis protocol.
9. Katie Leishman, "Mr. Catapano's Vaccine," *New York Native* (5/23/88): 19–24.
10. *Ibid*, 21.
11. *Ibid*, 19.
12. Dr. Harris L. Coulter, *op. cit.*, 43–46.

Chapter 4

The Forgotten Plague

And this disease of which I speak, this syphilis too will pass away and die out, but later it will be born again and be seen again by our grandchildren just as in bygone ages we must believe it was observed by our ancestors."

De Contagione—Girolamo Fracastoro[1]

The history of syphilis goes back almost as far as the recorded history of mankind. During that time, it has appeared under dozens of different names, and been manifested in innumerably different ways. More than anything else, the most consistent thing about syphilis has been its inconsistency.[2] It is a radical disease which under the right conditions knows no boundaries or rules, and it has been during those periods when we've attempted to make it fit into stereotypes that syphilis has done its worst damage.

There is no single, accepted history of syphilis upon which all historians agree. The main reason for this disagreement is the changing identity of the disease. The modern name, "syphilis," was first used by Girolamo Fracastoro (1483 – 1553) in his poem, "Syphilis Sive Morbus Gallicus," written in 1530. However, it would not be until the 1700s that this term would be internationally adopted.[3] In the meantime, syphilis went under dozens of different names, some of the most common being listed below:[4]

The French Disease (Italy)
The Neopolitan Evil (France)
The French Pox (Germany/England)
The Bordeaux Evil (Germany/England)
The Spanish Pox (Holland/N. Africa)
The Castilian Disease (Portugal)
The Christian Disease (Persia)
The Polish Disease (Russia)
The German Disease (Poland)

As may be evident, countries afflicted with syphilis were apt to blame the disease on nations or neighbors with whom they were in conflict. This was a likely development, as armies traveling to battle were the most common means by which syphilis was, and still is, spread across political borders.

In addition to multiple names, the manifestations of syphilis were for centuries poorly understood. It would not be until the writings of Philippe Ricord (1800 – 1889) and Jean Alfred Fournier (1832 – 1914) that syphilis would take on a recognizable definition. Until then, however, the signs and symptoms, and the names of the signs and symptoms, just like the name of the disease itself, changed from country to country and period to period. This has left historians with the daunting task of trying to determine the exact history of syphilis in man.

Given the problems they face, most historians today agree that the earliest writings on syphilis were those of the Chinese, some 2000 years before Christ. In 1863, Captain Darby's book, *La Medecine Chez Les Chinois*, was published in Paris. Darby travelled to the Orient and while there assembled a history of their medicine. Though, of course, the Chinese did not use our current name for the disease, Darby found manifestations in their ancient writings that were undeniably those of syphilis.[5]

In contrast to China, European history does not have records of syphilis prior to the 1400s AD. This has lead to what is called the "New World" theory of the origin of syphilis. The disease was absent from medical writings until shortly after Christopher Columbus returned from visiting Hispanola, part of which is known today as Haiti. Hispanola has historically been recognized as epidemic with syphilis. The New World theory postulates that Columbus and his crew brought the disease back to Europe upon returning from this island.[6] There is even evidence that Columbus himself died of syphilis infection.[7] After Columbus' return, medical literature about syphilis began to proliferate in Europe, as traveling armies spread the disease wherever they went. With respect to this, it is of interest to note the role Johannes Gutenberg (1397 – 1468), inventor of the first practical moving type printing press, played in the story of syphilis. Europeans of the 1400s were so desperate for information about this devastating new disease that authors of texts on syphilis were the first in history to have their books printed by press while they were still alive.[8]

In contrast to the New World theory is the Old World theory of the origin of syphilis. This second theory assumes syphilis to have been present and pathogenic in man for as long as homo sapiens have walked the earth. However, if the Old World version were correct, characteristic syphilitic bone lesions should have been found at anthropological dig sites in Egypt and Asia Minor. The notable absence of these lesions on recovered skeletal structures casts doubt upon this theory.[9] Also, the Old World theory does not explain why, if the disease has always been with us, there was the sudden epidemic in Europe of the 1400s. Unfortunately, neither of these two theories is comprehensive about the origins of syphilis, as the New World theory explains little of what happened before the 1400s. For this reason, many historians have sought a more comprehensive proposition that would include pre-Columbian history, like the writings of Darby, yet also account for the surges and recessions of syphilitic afflictions around the globe.

The deficiencies of the Old and New World theories have led to the development of a third concept: the Modified-Columbian theory. Syphilis is a disease of opportunity. Over time our bodies can become acclimated to this disease, though not totally immune to it. It is a process which can take decades or centuries, but an equilibrium between the body and the bacterium can be achieved. While undisturbed, this period of balance will see mostly minor manifestations of syphilis. In contrast to this, if Treponema pallidum (TP), the causative agent of syphilis, is introduced into a population of individuals who have not been previously infected, the disease will appear in its worst form possible: malignant syphilis.[10] In this form, the disease rampages through the body in an unpredictable and lethal manner. This was what happened to Europe in the 1400s.

Yet, within fifty years, Europeans had become adapted to the bacterium, and syphilis appeared in less virulent forms.[11]

Along with man's ability to adapt to the bacterium, TP can adapt to its environment. The Modified-Columbian theory assumes, like the Old World theory, that TP has been around probably as long as, if not longer than man. Like homo sapiens, the bacterium has spread across the globe, and, given the different environments in which it finds itself, has undergone subtle yet significant changes into a variety of different strains. This differentiation of TP into strains is analogous to mankind's differentiation into races: Negro, Oriental, Caucasian, etc. Yet, just as the color of a man's skin does not limit his potential for violence, each strain of TP retains specific abilities to cause disease. Syphilis had probably visited Europe long before the 1400s but, given time, the inhabitants there became acclimated to their particular strain of the bacterium. However, this did not guarantee their safety against the new strain of TP Columbus brought back from Hispanola. Thus, Europeans were attacked by a new "race" of TP; one to which they had not adapted. This was the basis for the epidemic of the 1400s. By the Modified-Columbian theory, syphilis has always existed, but is only manifested in its catastrophic malignant form when a new strain of TP is introduced into a population not previously infected by that strain. This malignant period will sooner or later give way to a period of acclimation and less virulent forms of the disease, until such time as another novel strain of TP arrives.[12]

Though syphilis has been consistently present in medical records since the 1400s, it took centuries for our understanding of the disease to become organized enough to postulate the Modified-Columbian theory. However, the path between the European epidemic and today has been slow and often misdirected. TP itself was not discovered until 1905. Therefore, much of this period was spent postulating explanations about the disease which were of little therapeutic value. Yet, hundreds of years of suffering were not totally wasted, as Phillipe Ricord, a Paris physician, established the foundations of our current understanding of the disease in the mid-1800s, even before TP was identified. Europe had over three centuries of recorded history with the bacterium by then yet, before Ricord, its manifestations were poorly understood and often confused with those of gonorrhea. Ricord made a definitive distinction between the two diseases, and even distinguished three stages of syphilis that, when non-malignant, the disease appears to follow. Jean Albert Fournier, a student of Ricord's, built upon his teacher's work, documenting syphilis' ability to leave its host open to infection by other degenerative diseases, the necessity for long-term therapy in treating the treponemal disease, and TP's role in congenital ailments. The work of these men organized the available knowledge of the nineteenth century into a system useful for the understanding and symptomatic treatment of syphilis. However, realistic attempts at curative treatment would have to wait for the discovery of the organism which actually caused the disease.

While our current understanding of syphilis began with the work of Ricord and Fournier,[13] they were unable to identify the microorganism which was responsible for the disease. By the time the gonococcus which causes gonorrhea was discovered in 1880 by Albert Neisser (1855 – 1916), most researchers believed that syphilis too had a microscopic component. In May of 1905, Fritz Schaudinn, a protozoologist, and Erich Hoffman, a syphilologist, discovered the bacterial origin Ricord could not find: TP.[14] Their identification of this organism paved the way for research into curative treatment of syphilis. It also enabled future researchers to further elaborate on the concepts originally established by the Parisians in the 1800s.

Treponema Pallidum is a bacterium classified by the following taxonomy.[15]

Order	:	Spirochaetales
Family	:	Spirochaetaceae
Genus	:	Treponema
Species	:	Pallidum

It is a corkscrew-shaped organism that ranges from 5 to 15 microns in length, and averaging from 0.1 to 0.15 microns in diameter.[16] It is a very active organism, whose ability for movement was highly appreciated shortly after its discovery. In 1936, Dr. Wm. A. Hinton of Boston wrote:[17]

> The motility of the T. Pallidum is somewhat characteristic and has been aptly described as that of an animated corkscrew. The organisms move chiefly in the direction of their long axis, transversing a straight or

an irregularly curved path with some rotary motion, as if they were actually screwing their way through the medium. A treponeme may curve slowly or quickly, forming small or large arcs of circles, or it may bend so sharply in the middle as to form a right angle and then rather quickly resume its original straight corkscrew shape.

Within 12 hours of infection by the organism, TP spreads rapidly throughout the body.[18] The blood and lymphatic circulatory systems carry it to virtually every bodily organ, including the central nervous system.[19] Long before the most commonly recognized first sign of the disease appears, a chancre at the site of initial infection, the bacterium has already traveled to every corner of the body.[20] However, once there, it does not stop. The bacterium not only wiggles and wriggles its way between each and every cell, but it actually moves into and invades bodily cells. This process, known as intracellularity, is thought to be responsible for the latency period found in the classical stages of non-malignant syphilis. The possibility that TP could attain intracellularity was raised a few months after its discovery. Since 1906, dozens of investigators have presented supportive evidence of the organism's capability. A 1975 researcher, T. J. Fitzgerald, found that intracellularity could be achieved as early as thirty minutes after infection.[21] Many other scientists had similar results,[22] with TP demonstrated to have entered a variety of cell types, including: [23]

plasma cells
fibroblasts
interstitial cells
Leydig cells
spermatocytes
neutrophils
macrophages
endothelial cells
perivascular connective tissue cells
epithelial cells

This ability of the Treponema pallidum to enter bodily cells has very serious consequences, which were summarized as follows in 1974: [24]

These findings of intracellular treponemas in human tissue cells lends emphasis to the suggestion of Sykes and Miller (1971) that intracellular organisms might be associated with the phenomena of latency. It is possible also that difficulties in treating effectively cases of human syphilis could be associated with the observed intracellular location of the treponemas which would render them inaccessible to humoral antibodies and to therapeutic substances.

Not only can the TP run rampant through an unsuspecting host, it can also hide inside their very cells, beyond the reach of natural antibodies and medicinal antibiotics. This capability of the bacterium has not been appreciated, as most physicians will state that the current penicillin therapy will cure treponemal infection. Unfortunately, they do not take into account the fact that while the first signs and symptoms of the disease may not appear for weeks, the organism may be hidden from therapeutic reach within hours. The penicillin may help eliminate the current manifestations a patient is suffering, but the TP remains latent, hiding and waiting.

Prior to the discovery of penicillin, syphilis used to be a critical area of medical study. From the 1500s through the 1940s, whole texts were devoted to the topic. General dermatology texts, which covered all skin ailments, often had one-quarter of their content devoted just to syphilis.[25] Today it is hard to find a medical book with more than ten to twenty pages on this subject. The disease is usually described, in modern texts, as following three specific stages during infection: primary, secondary, and tertiary. These stages are well defined in dozens of books [26] and will not be repeated here, for it is not the regular syphilis which should be of concern to us. It is malignant syphilis—which has not been seen on a massive scale since the epidemic of the 1400s, following no patterns or stages and seldom mentioned in today's medical texts—which is likely the actual cause of AIDS today.

Malignant syphilis is the form of this disease which appears in sudden epidemics when TP enters a population never before affected by the bacterium, or a new strain of the organism appears in a population previously afflicted with a different strain of TP. Under these conditions, the disease manifestations are erratic and unpredictable. Symptoms commonly thought to occur only in late tertiary stages of syphilis may appear in the first months, the patient appearing to have bypassed the symptomatology of the first and second stages. Rules of order are abandoned and often the ravaged patient will die within a year.[27]

This obscure form of the disease, about which few doctors have ever read, let alone seen, only occurs when a bacterial strain encounters a new host environment to infect. Yet, we and our immediate ancestors have been continually afflicted with syphilis since the 1400s. What has changed? The answer lies not in the bacterium, as was the case with Columbus, but with our own bodies. We have, through medical, social, and behavioral influences, become new environments for old strains of TP. Our bodies have literally gone through subtle, yet significant changes in their internal biochemical makeup and mechanisms, the most important of these changes occurring in our immune systems. To the treponemas, we have become new environments, waiting for the forgotten plague to appear once more.

The factors whose interaction allowed syphilis to become malignant are numerous and intricate. Current medicinal therapies like penicillin and other antibiotics have played a major role in setting the stage for disaster. They were believed to be curative, yet could only offer symptomatic relief which was often temporary. Certainly, one individual infected with syphilis and treated by this symptomatic regimen would not have been enough to start a malignant rampage. However, this factor was not operating alone. Freer sexual mores of the 1960s and 1970s allowed people to receive multiple infections with TP that, in turn, would be treated symptomatically with penicillin. Also, recreational drugs of all types were, and still are, commonly used by many people. These drugs wreak their own havoc on the immune system, which when added to multiple, ineffectively treated infections by TP, have prepared the way for tragedy. Our bodies were biochemically altered beyond the point of the balance so important to restricting syphilis to its classical stages. To the bacterium, we were a new host lacking the immunity of equilibrium which could prevent malignant manifestations of the disease.

Today, the efficacy of penicillin treatments for syphilis is waning. Our current rates of contagious syphilis infections are the highest since 1950, the beginning of the decade when penicillin became the main form of syphilis therapy.[28] The *New York Times* reported, in October of 1987, that "the number of syphilis cases has more than doubled in New York City, is up 97 percent in Los Angeles County, and has risen 86 percent in Florida, according to state and local officials." [29] These three areas happen to be those with the highest rates of AIDS, with the amounts of increase in syphilis cases corresponding to their respective number of AIDS cases. As would be anticipated, with more adults being infected with syphilis, there has also been a corresponding increase in the number of congenital cases of the disease.[30] Children too have suffered terribly from syphilis. Yet, the potential for such an outbreak was well-known long before AIDS appeared, as in 1974 a panel of experts organized by the U.S. Public Health Services, the World Health Organization, the Pan American Health Organization, and the International Union Against Venereal Disease and Treponematoses, concluded: [31]

> The participants of the seminar, in noting the rising trends in incidence of both syphilis and gonorrhea in the United States of America, are of the opinion that the medical, social, and behavioristic factors operating in modern society are likely to lead to a further increase in the prevalence of venereal diseases in the United States of America as well as in other countries throughout the world. Existing epidemiological and other methods have failed to control the spread of these diseases in and between countries in the United States of America as well as in other countries, and new approaches are therefore necessary.

Yet no new approaches have been taken. In fact, due to budget cuts, old approaches like the tracking of sexual contacts of known syphilitics have been abandoned.[32] This taking of two steps backwards, instead of a step forward, has combined with many other factors in a complex and intricate manner to create the disease we know as AIDS. Malignant syphilis once ravaged Europe as immunodeficiency now ravages us. An organism hidden in both our bodies and in time has taken advantage of a situation we have created. Perhaps our very survival into the future will depend upon remembering the past, so that we may stop reliving it.

References

1. Dr. Wilmer Cave Wright, trans., *Contagion, Contagious Diseases, and Their Treatment, by Girolamo Fracastoro, 1546* (G.P. Putnam's Sons: 1930), 144–147.
2. E.L. Keyes, M.D., *The Venereal Diseases* (William Wood and Co: 1880), 57.
3. S. William Becker, M.D., and Maximilian E. Obermayer, M.D., *Modern Dermatology and Syphilology* (J.B. Lippincott Co.: 1943), 1; Herman Goodman, M.D., *Notable Contributors to the Knowledge of Syphilis*, (Froben Press: 1944).
4. Dr. Wm. Van Wyck, *The Sinister Shepherd* (The Primavera Press: 1934), 1.
5. E.L. Keyes, *op. cit.*, 46; Dr. E. Lancereaux, *A Treatise on Syphilis Historical and Practical*, trans., G. Whitley, M.D. (The New Sydenham Society: 1868), 1:8.
6. Becker and Obermayer, *op. cit.*, 1.
7. H. Goodman, *op. cit.*, 13.
8. *Ibid*, 7.
9. Becker and Obermayer, *op. cit.*, 3.
10. E.L. Keyes, *op. cit.*, 55.
11. Wm. Allen Pusey, M.D., *Syphilis as a Modern Problem* (Chicago: A.M.A.: 1915).
12. *The Florida Anthropologist*, Florida Anthropological Society, Inc., vol. 25, no. 4 (Dec. 1972): 175.
13. Wm. Allen Pusey, *op. cit.*, 25–27.
14. *Ibid*, pp. 33–34.
15. Mandell, Douglas Jr., and Bennett, *Principles and Practices of Infectious Diseases* (John Wiley and Sons: 1979), 1821.
16. *Ibid* (2nd ed., 1985), 1323.
17. Wm. A. Hinton, M.D., *Syphilis and its Treatment* (The MacMillan Co.: 1936), 8.
18. Wm. A. Pusey, *op. cit.*, 75.
19. Becker and Obermayer, *op. cit.*, 672.
20. Wm. A. Hinton, *op. cit.*, 47; Joseph Earle Moore, M.D., *Penicillin in Syphilis* (Charles C. Thomas, Publisher: 1946), 223.
21. T.J. Fitzgerald, et. al., "Treponema pallidum (Nicholas strain) in tissue cultures: Cellular attachment, entry, and survival," *Infection and Immunity*, vol. 11 (1975): 1133.
22. V. Lauderdale and J.N. Goldman, "Serial ultrathin sectioning demonstrating the intracellularity of T. pallidum: An electron Micro-

scope study," *British Journal of Venereal Diseases*, vol. 48 (1972): 87–96.

23. J.A. Sykes, J.N. Miller, and A.J. Kalan, "Treponema pallidum within cells of a primary chancre from a human female," *British Journal of Venereal Diseases*, vol. 50 (1974): 42.
24. *Ibid*, 44.
25. Becker and Obermayer, *op. cit.*, 672.
26. P.D. Hoeprich, *Infectious Diseases* (Harper and Row: 1972).
27. Dr. Harris L. Coulter, *AIDS and Syphilis—The Hidden Link* (North Atlantic Books and Wehawken Book Company: 1987), 5.; E.L. Keyes, *op. cit.*, 46; Dr. E. Lancereaux, *A Treatise on Syphilis Historical and Practical*, trans., G. Whitley, M.D. (The New Sydenham Society: 1868), 1:100.
28. "Syphilis rate on the rise, minorities are hardest hit," Associated Press, Atlanta, *The Miami Herald* (8/19/88): 27A.
29. Robert Pear, "Sharp rise found in syphilis in U.S.," *The New York Times* (10/4/87): 1.
30. Rosemary Goudreau, "More babies born with syphilis," *The Miami Herald* (8/18/88): 1C.
31. *Today's VD Control Program* (The American Social Health Association: 1974), 70.
32. J.E. D'Eramo, Ph.D., "Targeted for Negligence: Why I Resigned From the New York City Health Department," *Christopher Street*, issue 122 (May 1988): 19.

Chapter 5

The Gift That Never Stops Giving

Contagion has this illness widely spread;
And, I feel sure, will farther spread it yet;
As in the fields one scabby sheep the flock
Destroys, and one infected pig the stock.

—Juvenal (60?–140?)
Satires, II.78 [1]

Syphilis is a communicable disease which occurs after the human body is infected with Treponema pallidum. While communicability offers the disease many means of spreading from person to person, it also places limitations upon these mechanisms. The most obvious of these limitations is that in order to catch syphilis, you must have some form of direct or indirect contact with someone already infected with the bacterium. Syphilis is not a spontaneous disease. It does not appear by immaculate infection, but only by contact with physiques bearing gifts.

There are three general pathways by which syphilis can be transmitted from one individual to another: congenital infection from mother to child, direct physical contact between two individuals, or by contact with certain bodily fluids from an infected individual.[2] These means of transmission have offered TP access to a continual source of new hosts to conquer and survive within. Syphilitics have efficiently spread the bacterium within their historical periods, and through the millenniums of time by giving the gift that never stops giving.

Though syphilis has ample means of transmission, it is produced by an incredibly delicate life-form. TP can flourish inside the human body, but is extremely fragile outside this host environment. The organism's weakness was summarized by Becker and Obermayer as follows, in 1943: [3]

> The spirochetes die very quickly after leaving the body, especially if they are allowed to dry out. Thus many avenues of spread, as seen in other diseases, are not open to them. Spirochetes do not persist for long periods in the dust as do tubercle bacilli. They are not waterborne, as are members of the typhoid-colon-bacillus group. The organisms do not contaminate and survive in foods as do food contaminating organisms. There is no known carrier of the spirochaeta pallida as there is for malaria, yellow fever, trypanosomiasis, and other infectious diseases.

These observations remain valid today, as transmission of TP is still restricted to the three methods listed above. Yet, these have not kept syphilis from becoming a national problem in many countries. Of these, most African nations and the United States have been particularly hard hit, with more reports of syphilis infection than any other countries.[4] It is not mere coincidence that these are also the areas hardest hit by the AIDS epidemic.

Syphilis and AIDS are both passed from person to person by the same methods and within the same restrictions. Like syphilis, AIDS does not happen by immaculate infection, but requires direct or indirect contact with an infected individual. Like syphilis, AIDS is not contracted by casual contact, contaminated food, or through external biological vectors like mosquitoes. Both diseases are spread by one of the three methods previously mentioned for syphilis. The most common examples of each of these are prenatal infection, sexual intercourse, and blood transfusions.

Possibly the most tragic syphilitics are those who are born with the disease. This type of transmission occurs when a woman who has syphilis passes the TP organism to her unborn child through the placenta. Due to asymptomatic infection, the disease can often go undetected in the mother, yet the child is seldom so fortunate. The results of prenatal contamination are devastating, as the unborn child has no effective immune response to mount against the invading bacterium. In 1922, Dr. B. P. Thom noted that "of all the still-births occurring each year, a most conservative estimate would be that one-half are caused by syphilis." [5] Though less common today, stillbirths are still a frequent outcome of congenital infection. The spectrum of congenital syphilis encompasses every sign and symptom imaginable, including ulcerations so severe that gaping holes appear where a nose and mouth should have been.[6] It is probably these more horrific congenital cases which have earned syphilis its infamous reputation. Fortunately, current treatment can usually offer successful relief of postnatal ailments. However, even with treatment, irreversible deafness, blindness, and scarring may remain as testament to the child's condition.[7]

Those of us fortunate enough to have escaped congenital syphilis are still at high risk of contracting the disease some time in our lives. More than any other means, sexual transmission of TP is the most common method of acquiring the disease. The TP spirochetes can be found in bodily fluids and cells (spermatozoa) which are often exchanged between sex partners. In the United States, sexual practices have left the homosexual community at particular risk.

The pre-AIDS period was a period of considerable homosexual repression expressed in many different ways, two of the most destructive forms concerning marriage and employment. It was not, and is still not acceptable or legal for homosexuals to marry one another and settle down as a family unit. The church is quick to point out that since in and of themselves they cannot produce offspring, a marital union of homosexuals would be an abomination before God. Somehow, this should not matter, for we supposedly live in nation founded upon the separation of church and state. More importantly, in a world with so many unwanted children, gay families could become a badly needed resource for those without parents. Still, moralists decry that gays are not to be trusted as parents for they would turn their young charges into homosexuals. This is not only unfounded speculation but a double standard also, as they don't dare apply the same reasoning to heterosexual families, from which all gays currently come. It is not surprising that the prejudice which denies gays legal rights to form families is so nonsensical. It is the product of homophobia which we socialize into our young at an early age, and most carry with them for the rest of their lives. Like other socialized phobias, the goal is repression, not logic, and repression starts at home with the family. Thus, gays have been denied the fundamental stability of this social unit in their adult lives.

Beyond the home, gays have faced, and still face repression in the work place. In many states, it is legal for an employer to fire an employee discovered to be homosexual, with our military one of the worst abusers of this form of repression. It is little wonder that homosexuals live such cloistered private lives. The stress of being denied a legal family unit to grow within, and the fear of losing employment have compromised the gay community into living double lives between their work and night life. During the day, an image of heterosexuality is the rule, but in the dark, the satisfaction of sexual relief, which the animal nature of all mankind demands, can be found. Homosexuals have settled for sexual relief, instead of love. Physical interaction has replaced the expression of emotional devotion which society has denied them. Relationships which could have offered healthier balances between physical and spiritual interactions have been pushed askew by the mores of our time.

For many gays of the late seventies and early eighties, sex became the cornerstone of socializing, with bathhouses serving as palaces of anonymous sex. While the rewards were high for those seeking release, so were the health risks. Sexual acts were developed which brought the most erogenous zones of the body—mouth, genitals, and anus—into close intimate contact. Fellatio (mouth-genitals), anilingus (mouth-anus), and anal intercourse (genitals-anus) offered a wide array of pleasure for the interested fun-seeker. But at the same time, sexual partners were exposed to multiple pathways for cross-infecting one another. These areas of pleasure are also three of the largest orifices of our bodies, each covered with sensitive mucous membrane. Passionate sexual interaction can often lead to small abrasions and, sometimes, bleeding cuts into these membranes, especially during anal intercourse. However, as noted by Becker and Obermayer in 1943, the spirochetes of TP can pass from one individual to another even in the absence of bleeding: [8]

> An element of considerable importance in infection with syphilis is that the two regions of the body where the organism grows best, namely the mouth and the genitalia, are lined and covered with mucous membranes or epithelium of the mucocutaneous junction, both of which are more delicate than the skin and more apt to be the seat of microscopic or macroscopic abrasions . . . Experiments have shown that the spirochete can pass through even normal mucosa . . . Neisser pointed out that trauma need only be sufficient to allow the organism to penetrate into lymphatic space, and that rupture of a blood vessel was not necessary.

This was written in the 1940s, when homosexual practices were not considered proper for medical discussion, let alone texts. Notably, it fails to mention the role anilingus and anal-intercourse may play in syphilis infection. However, today, as we progress to a more open and honest understanding of each other, the subject is beginning to be addressed, as in this example by Henry Masur and Abe Macher: [9]

> Specific sexual practices have a particularly important influence on the development of gastrointestinal infection and inflammation in homosexual men. Any practice that facilitates direct or indirect oral-rectal contact will enable rectal and fecal microorganisms to be ingested by the sexual partner . . . Genital-rectal sex followed by genital-oral sex, or genital-rectal intercourse with one partner followed by genital-rectal sex with another partner, allows the penis to serve as a vector for indirect transmission of enteric organisms.

Yet, before today's epidemic, there were other risks inherent in the gay lifestyle. Not only were the sexual practices themselves placing homosexuals at risk of syphilitic infection, but, as mentioned above, matters were made worse by practicing these sexual acts with more than one partner. This was often the case at bathhouses and backrooms, where a person could have multiple sexual contacts in the same evening, and then come back the next night to find all new people with whom to interact. Masur and Macher summed up this problem as follows: [10]

> Multiple sexual partners and anonymous sex also facilitates transmission of infection. The anonymity of sexual encounters makes it unlikely that a homosexual will have any knowledge of the health status of his partner or that his partner can be traced if the homosexual discovers that he has a sexually transmissible disease. Other major factors that complicate identification of infected individuals are the high frequency of asymptomatic rectal or oropharyngeal processes, such as gonorrhea, syphilis, and herpes simplex, and the lack of sophistication of many physicians in screening, diagnosing, and treating sexually transmissible diseases in homosexual men.

Deprived of a legal family unit and threatened with loss of employment, gays created a community that maximized sexual satisfaction as compensation for those pleasures and securities mainstream society denied them. Continually faced with a world which hates them for loving one another, their very survival has been dependent upon ingenuity and adaptation. It is not surprising, therefore, once the hazards of sexual transmission of AIDS were identified, that it has been the gay community, and not the heterosexual community, which has been so quick to adapt the new attitudes and behaviors necessary to reduce such risks. These behavioral changes, including the use of condoms and practicing safer sex, help protect gays from infection by TP and the development of AIDS. As rates of new infection drop for homosexuals, it was reported at the Fourth International Conference on AIDS, held June of 1988 in Stockholm, that the number of heterosexual AIDS cases is on the rise, and their "risk greatly increases if one of the partners has a venereal disease that causes genital ulcers, such as genital herpes, syphilis, or chancroid." [11] This situation parallels that for syphilis, as the *Communicable Disease Handbook*, published in 1982, states, "The male homosexual group in large cities is particularly at risk, followed by heterosexuals with multiple sexual partners." [12] Unfortunately, too many people in the United States continue to live under the illusion that syphilis is a curable, nearly non-existent disease, and AIDS is a gay disease. Perhaps it will only be after their ignorance has caused the same suffering and loss of life in their community, as it has in the gay community, that mainstream America will pay attention to a disease that is everyone's problem.

The third major pathway by which syphilis and AIDS are spread is through contact with bodily fluids from an infected individual. The most common example of this type of transmission is blood transfusion. It is in respect to this means of infection that the greatest myth about syphilis has been propagated. In 1977, the following statement appeared in the seventh edition of the American Association of Blood Banks' (AABB) technical manual: [13]

> Diseases such as malaria and syphilis can be transmitted by transfusion . . . Since the Treponemal spirochete does not survive seventy-two-hour refrigeration, fresh blood or other blood products such as platelet concentrations which are not stored refrigerated prior to use have the greatest risk of syphilis transmission.

In the eighth edition, published in 1981, this statement became: [14]

> The treponemal spirochete cannot survive at refrigerator temperature, so only products stored at room temperature or transfused very promptly after donation have any risk of syphilis transmission.

Meanwhile, in the ninth edition, published in 1985, the statement was revised to: [15]

> Transmission of syphilis by transfusion is possible, but requires that blood be drawn during the rather brief period of spirochetemia, and that the organisms remain viable at the time of transfusion. The treponemal spirochete cannot survive more than 72 hours at 4 C so only components stored at room temperature (platelet concentrate) or transfused very promptly after donation have any risk of transmitting syphilis.

There is a crucial deception present throughout these three editions, concerning TP's ability to survive cold temperatures and the use of refrigeration to kill the bacterium. To support their claim, regarding temperature, all three publications reference a 1969 article written by three prominent figures in the AABB: R.W. Chambers, H.T. Foley, and P.J. Schmidt. Their research, titled, "Transmission of syphilis by fresh blood components," appeared in the ninth volume of *Transfusion*, the official journal of the AABB. Contrary to the technical manual's statements, this article clearly states: [16]

> In the usual situation when infected human blood is stored at 5 C in citrate anticoagulant, infectivity is lost in 96 hours or less. The treponema is not viable after storage for a few days to few weeks at -10 C to -20 C. It is viable, however, when stored for extended periods at -45 C and is infectious for an indefinite period when stored at -78 C.

In black-and-white these three authors have clearly stated that as the temperature goes down, the longevity of TP increases, to the point that at -78 C it is viable indefinitely. Even as early as 1943, Becker and Obermayer noted that "it has been found that extreme cold will preserve S. pallidum [TP] in virulent form for a long time." [17] In 1944, a text on clinical syphilis states that "refrigeration is a much less efficient protection than is generally supposed, but [*sic*] survival of the organism after 96 hours at 5 C has been demonstrated." [18] The AABB's misinterpretation may be at the heart of a deadly error when other practices of the association are taken into account. The 1970 publication of the fifth edition of the *Technical Methods and Procedures of the AABB* declares that "freezing red blood cells for indefinite lengths of time for subsequent transfusion has become an accepted blood bank procedure." [19] The temperatures used for freezing are -80 C and -150 C, well below the point needed for indefinite viability of the bacterium. The AABB is claiming spirocheticidal effectiveness for a process which actually preserves the syphilis organism. Thus, up to and throughout the AIDS epidemic, our blood banks have been a potentially significant transmission medium for the contagion most likely responsible for this disaster: TP.

One group particularly threatened by these blood bank procedures are the hemophiliacs previously mentioned in the second chapter. Their infection via factor VIII was the declared reason why researchers eliminated anything but viruses from the list of potential causative agents of AIDS. They determined that nothing larger than a virus would pass through the filtration process used in making the factor VIII. Yet, as previously discussed, TP is flexible and small enough to pass through the same size filter pores as can retroviruses. Nowadays, lyophilized factor VIII is the most common form of the coagulant factor given to hemophiliacs. The method used to produce this type of factor VIII supposedly kills any bacterium present. However, through the mid-seventies, a different kind of factor VIII was given to hemophiliacs: cryoprecipitated factor VIII. The process used to make this type of coagulating factor takes between twenty-four and forty-eight hours, and is done at temperatures between 4 C and -70 C. [20] According to the article by Chambers, Foley and Schmidt, and contrary to the AABB technical manual, the TP is not killed by these temperatures during such short time frames. The old, pre-AIDS factor VIII was a potential storehouse for TP and would not prevent the hemophiliacs from catching syphilis or developing AIDS.

It is very likely that the practices of blood banks in the United States and elsewhere have not been protecting us from syphilis infection. The bactericidal claims of the AABB are not only unsupported by the very references they base their statements upon, but are actually contradicted by these references. The reasons for their actions, in the light of the health risks to which they are exposing blood transfusion recipients, are probably economical in nature. There are approximately three million blood transfusions annually in the U.S.[21] Of these, only a small percent are likely to be contaminated with TP. Therefore, the cost of testing all donor blood would be prohibitively expensive, as only a small percentage of transfusion recipients are statistically at risk of TP infection. Thus, the 1985 edition of their technical manual states the "AABB Standards has dropped the requirement for serological tests for syphilis (STS) on donor blood." [22] As would be expected, given the open door TP policy of our blood banks, a small percentage of hemophiliacs have come down with AIDS.

Another group at risk for syphilis blood transfusion, though not due to AABB practices, are intravenous drug users: individuals who inject substances directly into their circulatory system. Often the needles used for these injections are shared by many users, without proper cleansing between injections. This allows small, yet significant amounts of contaminated blood and other bodily fluids to pass from one person to another, via the hypodermic needle. The results of hypodermic transmission are atypical of syphilis infection, as outlined by Becker and Obermayer: [23]

> A well-known form of infection with asymptomatic onset is that produced by instrumental introduction of spirochetes directly into the blood stream. If this happens by the prick of a needle harboring spirochetes, a primary lesion will not form at the site of the puncture, and the infection is systemic from the start (syphilis d'emblee). This is especially frequent in patients who have received blood from a syphilitic donor . . . Stokes quotes Burbi as stating that the course of transfusion syphilis differs from ordinary syphilis in that lymphatic involvement is usually minimal, that the eruption begins on the limbs instead of on the trunk, and that the incubation period is shorter than in ordinary syphilis.

Thus, like the blood transfusion recipient, the drug user may receive syphilis infection without any signs or symptoms as warnings. This infection becomes systemic faster than infection by other means, and, therefore, the spirochetes will attain intracellularity much quicker. The needle, whether for legal transfusion or illicit drug use, offers TP the quickest pathway for invading the human body, without warning the individual of its presence.

Like syphilis, AIDS is spread by blood transfusion, sexual contact, and congenital infection. An uninfected individual may become infected by one or more of these methods, once or more than once in their lifetime. These pathways are not only identical for, but significant links between syphilis and AIDS: links critical to establishing them as one and the same disease.

References

1. Maurice B. Strauss, M.D., *Famous Medical Quotations* (Little, Brown and Co.: 1968), 147.
2. Mandell, Douglas Jr., and Bennett, *Principles and Practices of Infectious Diseases* (John Wiley and Sons: 1979), 1822; S. William Becker, M.D., and Maximilian E. Obermayer, M.D., *Modern Dermatology and Syphilology* (J.B. Lippincott Co.: 1943), 679.
3. S. William Becker, M.D., and Maximilian E. Obermayer, M.D., *Modern Dermatology and Syphilology* (J.B. Lippincott Co.: 1943), 679.

4. Renee Sabatier, *Blaming Others—Prejudice, race and worldwide AIDS* (New Society Publishers, The Panos Institute: 1988), 70–71; *Today's VD Control Program* (The American Social Health Association: 1974), 51.
5. B.P. Thom, M.D., *Syphilis* (Lea and Febiger, Philadelphia and N.Y.: 1922), 327.
6. G.H. Fox, A.M., M.D., *Photographic Illustrations of Cutaneous Syphilis* (E.B. Treat, N.Y.: 1881), plate XLVII.
7. I. Bobak, Ph.D., and M. Jensen, R.N, M.S, *Essentials of Maternity Nursing* (C.V. Mosby Co.: 1987), 1037–1039.
8. Becker and Obermayer, *op. cit.*, 680.
9. H. Masur and A. Macher, "Infections in Special Hosts: Infections in Homosexual Men"; Mandell, Douglas Jr., and Bennett, *Principles and Practices of Infectious Diseases* (John Wiley and Sons: 1979), 1667.
10. H. Masur and A. Macher, "Infections in Special Hosts: Infections in Homosexual Men."
11. Rosemary Goudreau, "AIDS on rise for high-risk heterosexuals," *The Miami Herald* (6/14/88): 1A.
12. L.C. Bennett, B.S.N., and S. Searl, M.S., *Communicable Disease Handbook* (John Wiley and Sons: 1982), 185.
13. *AABB Technical Manual*, 7th ed., American Association of Blood Banks (1977): 253.
14. *Ibid*, 8th ed. (1981): 318.
15. *Ibid*, 9th ed. (1985): 339.
16. R.W. Chambers, H.T. Foley, and P.J. Schmidt, "Transmission of Syphilis by Fresh Blood Components," *Transfusion*, vol. 9 (1969): 32.
17. Becker and Obermayer, *op. cit.*, 672.
18. Stokes, Beerman, and Ingraham, *Modern Clinical Syphilology*, 3rd ed. (W.B. Saunders Co.: 1944), 471.
19. *Technical Methods and Procedures of the AABB*, 6th ed., American Association of Blood Banks (1974): 220.
20. *Ibid*, 5th ed. (1970): 181–184.
21. Bob Stein, "AIDS risk from blood transfusion assessed," UPI (Boston), 2/24/88.
22. *AABB Technical Manual*, 9th ed., *op. cit.* (1985): 339.
23. Becker and Obermayer, *op. cit.*, 680.

Chapter 6

Seeing Is Believing

To know syphilis is to know medicine.
—Sir William Osler[1]

With venereal diseases, the exact means by which any particular individual becomes infected is often questionable. Usually, the onset of symptoms occurs long after infection. Such is the case with both syphilis and AIDS. Ultimately the issue of who gave what to whom is secondary to the question of whether or not disease is present, a question answered by signs and symptoms. Though the means of infection may be unclear, once identifiable manifestations of illness do appear, the fact that disease is present becomes undeniable. Seeing is believing.

While syphilis and AIDS do share the exact same modes of transmission, this alone does not prove them to be synonymous. Many organisms are spread by these means, so much so that simultaneous infection by two or more of them often occurs. However, though diseases other than syphilis are transmitted the same as AIDS, only TP is known to cause the exact same pathology as AIDS.

Syphilis, historically, has been shown to produce directly, or via secondary infections, almost every disease manifestation known to man. This chameleon quality is the basis of its nickname: the great imitator. The pathology produced by TP is so extensive, that all surfaces and "virtually any organ in the body can be involved." [2] This coincides with a similar statement about AIDS, in which "virtually every organ system is a potential target." [3]

Syphilis affects every organ and tissue of the body. Today, medical texts limit the progression of infection to three specific stages. The first of these stages occurs during the early months after infection, and is noted by a temporary chancre at the site of initial infection. Shortly after this primary stage, a secondary stage occurs, characterized by a body rash which also disappears in a matter of weeks or months. Then an asymptomatic period of latency is entered and may last for the remainder of an individual's life. However, it is possible, after latency begins, for the third or tertiary stage of syphilis to appear. It is this stage, in classical syphilis, where everything from the scalp to the toes is afflicted. Yet, when syphilis becomes malignant, the signs and symptoms obey no rules, and the classical stages become useless as diagnostic tools. Therefore, the important thing to remember is the pathology, irrespective of the expected chronology.

Prior to penicillin, syphilis was a significant topic in medical literature. However, after the advent of the antibiotic age, it was demoted from the subject of whole texts to the subject of a single chapter within texts on infectious diseases or dermatology. Nowadays, syphilis may not even receive that much attention and only be a subtopic within a chapter. It is truly a shame that such a shallow perspective is presented to today's clinicians concerning one of the greatest masqueraders of all time. Modern writings of syphilis depict it as a disciplined, structured adversary, rather than the ruthless killer it can be. Since the coming of penicillin, we have been slowly lulled into a false sense of security, of which malignant syphilis is now taking advantage.

Today, only older texts dating back before 1950 remain as testament to the terror and tragedy of syphilis. They are overflowing with records and references to the infinite spectrum of ailments which this disease can produce. As is expected by the syphilis theory, these older texts are incredibly similar to today's AIDS literature, the only difference being the choice of words used to name the disease. One of these, *The Practice of Urology—A Surgical Treatise on Genito-Urinary Disease Including Syphilis*, written in 1913, serves as a particularly good example. In its index under the heading "syphilis" and subheading "areas affected," the author, Dr. Chetwood, lists the following: [4]

alimentary tract	joints	pancreas
aponeuroses	kidney	pharynx
arteries	larynx	prostate
bladder	liver	rectum
bones	lungs	respiratory tract
bronchi	mouth	skin
bursae	mucous membrane	spleen
circulatory system	muscles	tendons
ear	nails	testicles
eye	nervous system	tongue
genito-urinary organs	nose	trachea
hair		

Other medical texts add to Chetwood's list by including mammary glands, digestive tract, esophagus, stomach, intestine, peritoneum, abdominal glands, ligaments, and cartilage.[5] These early twentieth century authors make the breadth of syphilis' symptomatic spectrum very clear: a spectrum equal to that seen in today's epidemic. As with AIDS, no part of our anatomy is safe when TP roams within us.

Once the bacterium of malignant syphilis goes on the offensive, it not only attacks everywhere, but in every way imaginable.[6] The skin can become victim to alopecia, rashes, and eruptions of condyloma, while mucous patches and ulcers erode the mouth. Generalized lymphadenopathy, fever, malaise, anorexia, and arthritis weaken the host's overall condition, while pharyngitis, laryngitis, glomerulonephritis, nephrotic syndrome, and hepatitis do more specific damage. Soon, the devastating symptoms of neurosyphilis may appear, including aphasia, ataxia, bladder disturbances, cranial nerve involvement, cerebral congestion, decreased memory, encephalitis, epilepsy, facial paralysis, hemiplegia, hyperactive reflexes, insanity, locomotor ataxia, meningitis, optic atrophy (blindness), paraplegia, peripheral neuropathy, sensorium (dementia), shooting pains, seizures, and stroke.[7] As in AIDS, malignant syphilis places no restrictions on when these ailments appear or how often they recur.

Like syphilis, the signs and symptoms of AIDS seem to be endless, as each year new manifestations are added to the list.

A whole book could be devoted to discussing the common pathology of the two diseases, but, within the scope of this text, detailed information will only be presented on the most prominent ailments. Some early manifestations will first be described, followed by intermediate and terminal inflammations and infections.

Fever, body rash (see above for syphilis), and swollen glands are three very common signs associated with AIDS. Historically, they and other AIDS manifestations have had a much longer connection to syphilis. In 1880, Dr. E.L. Keyes wrote that "all descriptions of syphilis, from the earliest times, have referred to fever as being one of the accompaniments of the disease." [8] Earlier, in 1814, Dr. Benjamin Bell noted that "this fever is always of the hectic kind, and accompanied with some colliquative symptom, particularly with nocturnal sweats." [9] Today, we know of many AIDS patients, present and past, drenched by feverish night sweats.

More than any other early warning sign, generalized lymphadenopathy is a hallmark of oncoming immunosuppression. Yet, swollen glands have long been recognized as symptomatic of syphilis also. In 1904, Dr. Edgar Ballenger commented that these glands "are firm, hard, non-inflammatory, freely movable, painless, and rarely suppurate [discharge pus]." [10] While crucial to the diagnosis of AIDS, this and other early signs were first known to those with syphilis.

Though AIDS and syphilis share characteristic early pathology, definitive clinical diagnosis of either is usually dependent upon further degenerative complications. These include dramatic weight loss, alopecia (baldness), loss of vision, and dementia. As is expected, each of these is intimately connected to syphilis. Of the weight loss, Bell wrote: [11]

> One of the most frequent symptoms of the advanced stages of syphilis is atrophy, or a gradual wasting of the body. From a state of obesity, and with a healthy, florid complexion, a person will in some instances become suddenly lean, while his face will be wan or sallow, as if vessels were altogether deprived of red blood. This I consider as one of the most fatal symptoms of the disease, from which, in the course of my observation few or none have ever recovered.

Along with this untimely loss of weight, Bell also found that alopecia may be the result of syphilis.[12] Keyes agrees with this and writes that it is possible syphilis "causes the shedding of all hair." [13] Added to the above, many AIDS patients also lose their ability to see. Bell concludes that: [14]

> . . . but in [syphilis], loss of vision to a considerable extent, has commonly taken place long before much pain is experienced; and if inflammation ever occurs, it is not in any remarkable degree. In some cases it comes on in a gradual manner. The sight becomes less perfect from day to day; and both the patient and friends are surprised that this should happen while the external appearance of the eye is not affected. But for the most part the disease takes place almost instantaneously, the patient being entirely deprived of vision in the course of a minute or two from the time the eyes become uneasy. In some cases only one eye is affected, but for the most part the disease attacks both at the same time.

Even children are not immune from syphilitic blindness, as Dr. David Nabarro notes in 1954 that congenital infection "may result in complete blindness in a considerable number of patients." [15]

Of all the losses suffered by AIDS patient's, dementia, loss of one's mind, is probably the worst. When this occurs along with physical degeneration, complete destruction of both body and soul are ensured. Dementia has been long recognized as characteristic of syphilis too.[16] It was, and still is, so prevalent in the United States that in 1938 Dr. Thomas Parran, then honorary chairman of the American Association for the Advancement of Science, estimated that the cost of hospital care for syphilis induced mental disorders was over thirty million dollars.[17] By 1976, this figure had increased to over sixty million dollars.[18]

Today, as with syphilis past and present, AIDS exacts a high price upon society. All of us are affected by it, yet it is the patients who suffer most. Multiple infections and afflictions are constant reminders of their plight, with Kaposi's sarcoma (KS), Pneumocystis carinii pneumonia (PCP), and thrush being three of the most common and definitive signs of AIDS.

Yet before today's epidemic, they were first associated with syphilis.

Moritz Kaposi (1837 – 1902) was a well renowned nineteenth century dermatologist from Vienna. He published papers on all aspects of skin diseases, and was a featured contributor to the European medical journal *Archiv fur Dermatologie und Syphilis* for thirty consecutive years. Many of his writings concerned syphilis,[19] though in 1872, his first paper published in the journal was about KS, which he called idiopathic multiple pigmented sarcoma.[20] Kaposi supposedly "first discovered the sarcoma lesions in syphilis patients," [21] though a recent translation of his original work contained no mention of this. Such an omission is not surprising, as the thesis of his paper was the sarcoma itself, and he may not have even made the connection between it and the treponemal disease at that time. Like syphilis, the sarcoma was known by many different names, with Kaposi changing it twice himself, and others contributing over thirty variations. It would not be until 1912, ten years after Kaposi's death, that the sarcoma would become a memorial to its discoverer.[22]

Historically, KS has long been associated with syphilis. As with TP, Becker and Obermayer note that KS "may affect almost every organ of the body." [23] One case study they use to depict typical KS is of a man previously infected with syphilis. This particular patient is considered exemplary of KS, as this case has been repeatedly used in description of the sarcoma.[24] Like syphilis, KS's severity of manifestation may be from the more benign to the "malignant form, death occurring in the latter in the course of a year of [*sic*] eighteen months, and even earlier." [25]

Pneumonias, as well as sarcomas, have been consistent and continuous manifestations of syphilis. Victor Cornil, author of a text on syphilis, wrote in 1882: [26]

> Syphilitic lesions of the lungs develop very insidiously, and may have reached a decided development while yet the symptoms are obscure. The symptoms are slight trouble in respiration, mild cough, often dry, and if expectoration exits, it is scanty and of the catarrhal kind . . . Later the symptoms become more marked, a severe form presenting all the features of well-developed consumption.

Today, like pneumonia itself, the dry, unproductive cough has become synonymous with AIDS. More specifically, PCP, the leading cause of death for AIDS patients, is known to occur after immunosuppression appears. The Pneumocystis organism responsible for the pneumonia, named after Dr. Carinii in 1912,[27] is commonly found among the many lung flora continually present in our bodies. Normally these organisms do not harm us, as our immune system maintains an equilibrium of checks and balances between our well being and their existence. However, when the immune system fails, as in chemoimmunosuppression for surgery patients, or due to infectious diseases like AIDS, this microbe can become a sure killer.

Syphilis too has been demonstrated to be a precursor for PCP. The 1976 paper titled "Pulmonary Pneumocystosis in Nonhuman Primates," [28] by F.W. Chandler of the CDC, discussed four cases of primate deaths due to this pneumonia. Two of the animals were owl monkeys who had been kept together in a cage several weeks before clinical signs of PCP appeared. Four years prior to this, one of them had been inoculated with TP, the equivalent of direct intravenous infection. The syphilis organism was the only clinical anomaly present in the medical history of either of the monkeys. Though both were males, there is nothing presented by the researchers which rules out homosexual transmission of TP from the infected to the uninfected monkey, just as it is seen in man. Treponemal infections are known to produce pneumonias, with this study being the first to demonstrate PCP as secondary to syphilitic infection.

Though not lethal as are PCP and KS, oral thrush is as significant and common a sign associated with AIDS, and syphilis. Like PCP, however, thrush, which is caused by the microorganism Candida albicans, is an opportunistic secondary infection. This was explained in the 1972 edition of the *Textbook of Dermatology*, as follows: [29]

> There is little evidence to indicate that C. albicans can become established as a pathogen in its own right in healthy individuals or tissues . . . Its establishment depends on the presence of some underlying pathological condition or other predisposing factor . . . So remarkably is C. albicans adapted to the exploitation of states of metabolic imbalance, that overt candidiasis should

> be regarded as the earliest manifestation of some more fundamental primary disorder.

Indeed it is well accepted today that thrush is one of the key diagnostic tools in evaluating AIDS patients. This is done by a process known as differential diagnosis, in which the immediate pathology is recognized as a side-effect of some underlying, more-fundamental illness. Though long forgotten, in 1939 Dr. H.M. Robinson, in his text *Practical Dermatology and Syphilis*, noted that the presence of thrush is an indication for a differential diagnosis of syphilis.[30] In addition, the presence of C. albicans often occurs simultaneous with that of oral leukoplakia[31] which is clinically indistinguishable from a type of thrush called chronic hyperplastic oral candidiasis.[32] One of the last and most definitive texts on the subject, *Modern Clinical Syphilology*, by Stokes, et. al., states: [33]

> On finding leukoplakia, look backward toward syphilis, forward toward cancer. Leukoplakia is not always of syphilitic origin, but it should always arouse a strong suspicion of syphilis.

As proper as it was for leukoplakia when originally written in 1944, today this quote applies just as well to thrush and the other symptoms of AIDS.

While it is beyond the scope of this text to review all AIDS pathology in detail, an undeniable similarity exists between it and syphilis. Though not explored here, it should be noted that TP, the microorganism responsible for syphilis, is "indistinguishable by known morphological, chemical, or immunological means from T. pertenue, T. carateum, or T.P. var Bosnia, which cause yaws, pinta, and endemic syphilis respectively." [34] These three latter diseases are merely different expressions of the same organism, and they represent all new areas of comparison between the width and breadth of TP and AIDS pathologies. Perhaps in an age full of new spirochetal diseases such as Lyme disease, TP will add to its credit a fifth face: AIDS.

References

1. Ebbesen, Biggar, and Melbye, *AIDS—A Basic Guide for Clinicians* (W.B. Saunders Co.: 1984), 56.
2. Mandell, Douglas Jr., and Bennett, *Principles and Practices of Infectious Diseases* (John Wiley and Sons: 1979), 1826.
3. Ebbesen, et. al., *op. cit.*, 56
4. C.H. Chetwood, M.D., *The Practice of Urology—A Surgical Treatise on Genito-Urinary Disease including Syphilis* (William Wood and Co, N.Y.: 1913), 811–812.
5. E.L. Keyes, M.D., *The Venereal Diseases* (William Wood and Co: 1880), 174–204, 218–230.
6. Mandell, et. al., *op. cit.*.
7. E.L. Keyes, *op. cit.*, 205–218.
8. *Ibid*, 101.
9. Dr. Benjamin Bell, *Treatise on Gonorrhoea and Lues Venerea* (E.F. Backus, Albany: 1814), part 2, 84.
10. Edgar G. Ballenger, M.D., *Genito-Urinary Disease and Syphilis* (E.W. Allen and Co, Georgia: 1908), 229.
11. Dr. Benjamin Bell, *op. cit.*, 83.
12. *Ibid*, 75–76.
13. E.L. Keyes, *op. cit.*, 172–173.
14. Dr. Benjamin Bell, *op. cit.*, 77.
15. David Nabarro, M.D., *Congenital Syphilis* (Edward Arnold, Ltd.: 1954), 328.
16. P.S. Sorensen and A.M. Nordenbo, "Neuro Syphilis in Greater Copenhagen Denmark During the Five Year Period 1974–1978," *Ugeskrift For Laeger* (1981): 2218.
17. F.R. Moulton, *Syphilis* (The Science Press: 1938), 192.
18. *VD Fact Sheet 1976*, 33rd ed., United States Public Health Services and the Center for Disease Control (1976): 3.
19. L.D. Bulkley, A.M., M.D., *Syphilis in the Innocent* (Bailey and Fairchild, New York: 1894), 311.
20. M. Kaposi, "Idiopathisches multiples Pigmentsarkom der Haut.," *Archiv fur Dermatologie und Syphilis*, vol. 4 (1872): 265–273.
21. Katie Leishman, "The AIDS Debate That Isn't," *The Wall Street Journal* (2/26/88): 21.
22. S.W. Becker and H.W. Thatcher, "Multiple Idiopathic Hemorrhagic Sarcoma of Kaposi: historical review, nomenclature, theories relative to nature of disease, with experimental studies of two cases," *Journal of Investigative Dermatology*, vol. 1 (1938): 379–398.
23. S. William Becker, M.D., and Maximilian E. Obermayer, M.D., *Modern Dermatology and Syphilology* (J.B. Lippincott Co.: 1943), 620.
24. Becker and Thatcher, *op. cit.*.
25. M.B. Hartzell, M.D., *Diseases of the Skin* (J.B. Lippincott, Co.: 1919), 621.

26. Victor Cornil, *Syphilis*, Victor Cornil, translated by Drs. Sims and White (Henry C. Leas's Son and Co., Philadelphia: 1882).
27. F.W. Chandler, H.M. McClure, W.G. Campbell, Jr. and J.C. Watts, "Pulmonary Pneumocystosis in Nonhuman Primates," *Arch. Pathol. Lab. Med.*, vol. 100 (1976): 163–167.
28. *Ibid.*
29. A. Rook, et. al., *Textbook of Dermatology*, 2nd ed. (Blackwell Scientific Publications: 1972): 759–760.
30. H.M. Robinson, M.D., *Practical Dermatology and Syphilis* (P. Blackison's Son and Co., Philadelphia: 1939), 321.
31. A. Rook, *op. cit.*, 1704.
32. *Ibid*, 762.
33. Stokes, Beerman, and Ingraham, *Modern Clinical Syphilology*, 3rd ed. (W.B. Saunders Co.: 1944), 729.
34. Holmes, Mardh, Sparling, and Wiesner, *Sexually Transmitted Diseases* (McGraw-Hill Book Co.: 1984), 291.

Chapter 7

The Blind Leading The Blind

We understand that a researcher on the West Coast is calling for Congress to grant amnesty to all doctors who have failed to diagnose AIDS correctly as syphilis. I think that such a move is wrong. All the AIDS patients who died because they were not correctly treated for syphilis deserve more than just a quilt in their memories. Their lovers and families deserve millions of dollars in compensation for this major episode of medical malpractice. I hope our readers will write to their congressional representatives and demand a vote of no on any proposals for syphilis amnesty.

—Charles L. Ortleb, N.Y. *Native*[1]

Though syphilis and AIDS share the same modes of transmission and the same signs and symptoms, many more years of experience exist diagnosing the former. However, the methods which we have relied upon for decades to determine the presence of TP are woefully inadequate and unreliable. More often than not, diagnosis has been misdiagnosis where syphilis is concerned. The inability to see and understand the cause of our illness has contributed to the epidemic spread of this disease.

Syphilis is one of the most universal infections known to mankind. It is found in every race, every country, and every socioeconomic group, regardless of political or religious affiliations. Yet, its universality is often disguised due to diagnostic difficulties. Just as the TP organism cannot be seen by the naked eye, physicians often misinterpret gross clinical manifestations which are tell-tale signs of syphilis. In addition, blood tests, which are supposed to be the safety net for patients not caught by clinical diagnosis, often do not detect the presence of TP. Thus, the afflicted entrust their health to those just as blind to their syphilitic infection as they are.

Clinical manifestations offer the first warnings of syphilis. In the classical stages, the first sign to appear is a painless chancre at the site of initial infection. Most people believe that this chancre appears only on the genitals but this is not true. It takes at least three weeks for the chancre to appear, from the onset of TP invasion.[2] This allows adequate time for the organism to circulate and attain intracellularity throughout the body, including the central nervous system. When the chancre finally appears, its location may be other than would be expected, as is described in the 1979 text *Principles and Practices of Infectious Diseases*: [3]

> The chancre is located wherever the inoculation takes place. The external genitalia are most frequently involved. Primary sites that are commonly overlooked are the cervix, mouth, perianal area, and anal canal in the females, and the perianal area, anal canal, and mouth of the male homosexual.

Dr. Henry H. Hazen preceded this with a more detailed list, in his 1915 text *Diseases of the Skin*, by noting the primary chancre of syphilis may appear on the lip, tongue, tonsil, gums, soft palate, buccal side cheeks, chin, cheeks, eyelid, nose, forehead, scalp, arm and hand, anus, breast, trunk, legs, and neck.[4] While the mode of transmission helps to determine if and where the chancre will manifest itself, every inch of the outer body and some inside the body are potential targets. As noted in chapter five, in the case of infection via blood transfusion, no chancre even appears. The chancre may also be missing if an individual receives antibiotics for reasons other than syphilis within a week or two of initial TP infection. These antibiotics, which are often given for other simultaneous venereal infections such as gonorrhea, suppress manifestation of the syphilis chancre.[5] Stokes, et. al, noted in 1944, that a method is needed "which will keep the masked syphilis from slipping through, to go on to infectious relapse and recurrence." [6] Such a method has never been developed. However, many times when a chancre does manifest, it is never detected due to its location and painless nature, especially anal and cervical chancres. Therefore, syphilis may be easily misdiagnosed or not even noticed by a patient or clinician who only relies upon genital chancres for positive identification.

The next most notable warning of early TP infection is the body rash associated with the second stage of classical syphilis. Whereas the chancre may avoid diagnosis or be misdiagnosed due to its location, the proper diagnosis of syphilitic rash is hampered by its multitude of atypical manifestations. Dr. W.A. Hinton, of Boston, wrote in 1936: [7]

> From the variety and distribution of cutaneous lesions of the secondary stage it is easy to see how the rashes of syphilis may be confused with those of many other diseases, chief among which are ringworm, tinea versicolor, pityriasis, rosea, psoriasis, erythema multiforme, seborrheic dermatitis, measles, German measles, severe acne, impetigo contagiosa, scabies, lichen planus, smallpox, tuberculosis, leprosy, yaws, chronic urticaria, scarlet fever, and rarely typhoid fever (particularly because of its "rose spots").

Given the difficulty in accurately diagnosing syphilis via chancre and rash, Hinton went on to state that "in possibly a third or even a half of the cases with manifest tertiary syphilis, the most careful clinical examinations have not revealed evidence of either of these early manifestations." [8]

Beyond these two landmarks of syphilis, the clinical diagnosis of TP infection becomes increasingly confused as the disease progresses. Among other things, it may be confused for acute meningitis, sensorineural hearing loss, iritis, anterior uveitis, optic neuritis, Bell's palsy, gastropathy, proctitis, hepatitis, pulmonary infiltration, nephrotic syndrome, glomerulonephritis, periostitis, tenosynovitis, polyarthritis, or infectious mononucleosis.[9] A 1977 article in the *Archives of Internal Medicine* reported on five cases where syphilis was misdiagnosed as cancer. Four of these five were seen at the Memorial Sloan-Kettering Cancer Center, where three of them were being considered for either radical surgery or extensive radiation and/or chemotherapy, before the proper diagnosis of syphilis was made. In the words of the article's authors, "failure to make an appropriate diagnosis in these patients could have had serious consequences." [10]

The inability of physicians to properly diagnose syphilis was underlined by a 1981 *Journal of the American Medical Association* article titled "Physician Recognition of the Signs and Symptoms of Secondary Syphilis." The author, Dr. Thomas Chapel of Wayne State University, Detroit, found that over sixty percent of the physicians in his study were unable to make a correct primary diagnosis of syphilis. He commented that "the data from this study show that physicians must not become complacent but remain alert for the physical and serological evidence of infectious syphilis." [11] Obviously, there is much syphilis out there which has been misdiagnosed. Yet, the problem of undetected syphilis is not unique to the United States. A 1973 article in the *British Journal of Venereal Diseases* notes that in England, "the incidence of undiscovered syphilis in any year during the period 1931 – 70 was of the order of 70 percent in the case of males and 100 percent in the case of females of the first-year infections discovered in that year." [12]

The most distressing cases of syphilis misdiagnosis involve its alter ego: AIDS. As noted in the opening quote of this chapter, many cases of syphilis are being misinterpreted, and subsequently mistreated, under current AIDS guidelines. A 1984 case report in the *North Carolina Medical Journal* is a prime example of this. The patient had many of the classical signs and symptoms of AIDS, including swollen lymph glands, night sweats, nausea, vomiting, anorexia, weight loss, fever, headaches, bodily rashes, and lesions. Fortunately, however, the authors, of Duke University Medical Center, were ultimately able to correctly diagnose "secondary syphilis masqueraded as AIDS in this patient." [13] In 1986, a similar case of near misdiagnosis in a female was reported in the November issue of *Hospital Practice*.[14]

One of the key problems in spotting TP infection concerns the serological laboratory tests used to aid diagnosis. Today, the two most commonly used blood tests are of the nontreponemal type: they react to the presence of bodily tissue changes related to but not specific for TP.[15] They do not directly react to the treponeme itself, with these tissue reactions often due to factors other than the bacterium. For this reason, they are also called non-specific serum tests, the two most widely used of these being the Venereal Disease Research Laboratory slide test (VDRL), and the Rapid Plasma Reagin test (RPR). Both are fairly inexpensive and provide quick results, but they are unreliable in detecting advanced forms of syphilis: forms seen in the later years of classical TP infection or in the first few years of malignant syphilis.

Non-specific tests have won their popularity due to their quick and inexpensive ability to detect early primary syphilis.[16] This is the type of TP infection for which a chancred-penis-bearing patient goes to the doctor three weeks after the fact. However, as noted, it is possible for early classical signs to go entirely unnoticed or not appear at all. By the time a patient reaches the doctor, his or her manifestations may be of well-advanced syphilis, which in the case of malignant infection may take less than a year to develop.

The most widely publicized defect of nontreponemal tests is that they react to changes in bodily tissue which can be caused by things other than the TP bacterium. Thus, individuals may be incorrectly diagnosed as having syphilis, when in fact they do not. However, of greater concern is the individual who has syphilis but whose blood tests are negative. While false-positives may cause undue concern and result in unnecessary prophylaxis, the syphilitic unwittingly convinced he is not infected is in far more serious danger. The VDRL and RPR are notoriously unreliable in detecting advanced or malignant syphilis. These tests, which rely on normal tissue immune responses are totally defeated when alterations in the immune system occur due to TP infection. As early as 1943, Becker and Obermayer were reporting cases of seronegative individuals in which "the presence of a negative [serum test] reaction in such patients may be explained on the basis of the blocking of antibody production by an overwhelming infection (Kahn) . . . treatment is followed by normal production of antibodies and a subsequent reversal of the test."[17] More recently, a study released in 1969 by Dr. J. Lawton Smith of Miami, shows the VDRL detected only thirty-two percent of the patients with advanced syphilitic infection, with over half of those detected showing only weak serum test reactions.[18] While the patients showed many signs of TP infection, nearly 70 percent of them had no tissue response for the VRDL to find. According to the *Princi-*

ples and Practices of Infectious Diseases, the RPR is even less reliable in detecting these advanced cases.[19] A 1964 article in the *Journal of the American Medical Association* warned of this, by stating: [20]

> Blind reliance on standard serological test for syphilis may be misleading. In our study, the disease, in various stages, was present in 24 patients whose serological tests were negative.

This warning echoes that of Becker and Obermayer, who were able to recognize this detrimental habit in the early 1940s: [21]

> At the present time, undue emphasis is often placed on laboratory procedures in all branches of medicine. In former times a physician had to spend many years perfecting himself at the art of clinical syphilology before he could attempt to care for a patient with syphilis. At present, it is the unfortunate belief of many physicians that it is only necessary to produce blood for the serological reaction, and, if positive, to start treating the patient without further examination.

These tests have such notorious reputations that by 1981 the American Association of Blood Banks, who previously had recommended the use of the RPR and other syphilis screening tests, "dropped the requirement for serological tests for syphilis (STS) on donor blood." [22] However, the federal government still mandates STS testing of donor blood, with the VDRL and RPR being the two most popular screening tests.[23]

There are other more advanced serum tests for detecting syphilis infection. Two of these, the Fluorescent Treponemal Antibody Absorption (FTA-ABS) and the Microhemagglutination Treponema pallidum (MHA-TP) are specific treponemal tests. Unlike the VDRL and RPR, these tests detect the presence of antibodies produced exclusively for defense against TP.[24] They are much more reliable in cases involving advanced syphilitic infection. However, due to their expense, most laboratories only use them to verify a positive VDRL or RPR test. Syphilis which may have been detected by the FTA-ABS or MHA-TP may never undergo these tests as a preliminary VDRL or RPR may unwittingly stop further investigation.

Overall, serological testing for syphilis is in a sad state of affairs. With many physicians lacking the expertise to properly diagnose clinical landmarks of TP infection, their overreliance on inexpensive and unreliable laboratory tests places the syphilitic at substantial risk of misdiagnosis. When a 1986 article in the British medical journal *Lancet* reported three AIDS cases in which all the patients had a history of syphilis, but were seronegative for TP infection, the diagnostic focus became viral. Given their symptoms included headaches, body rashes, fever, swollen lymph glands, and thrush, all known manifestations of the bacterium, a differential diagnosis of advanced syphilis was notably absent. While the article's authors were quick to point out that "the characteristic skin eruption, which mimics roseola, may be a dermatological marker of acute HTLV-III infection," [25] they blatantly ignored the fact that roseola is "a rose-colored rash, as may be seen in measles, syphilis, and certain other exanthematous diseases." [26] Unfortunately, the actual role TP played in these patients' illness may never be known, due to research efforts thwarted by unreliable serum tests. This problem was foreseen by Dr. J.A. Kolmer in 1928 when he noted that "the important lesson to be learned by the majority of practitioners is not to ignore positive reactions but to distrust negative reactions and never to accept a single negative as excluding syphilis when suspicious clinical signs or history are present." [27]

Today, the accurate diagnosis of syphilis is doubtful, due to missing or misinterpreted clinical signs and questionable laboratory tests. What is perceived as an easily detectable illness is quite capable of slipping by clinicians and technicians alike. An infected individual may be allowed to pass his disease on to countless others, all under the seal of approval from his local physician. In addition, infected individuals may pass TP on to each other, thus compounding their original infection, further increasing the potential for malignant outbursts. AIDS appeared on the heels of two decades of sexual experimentation. It was a time of unhindered and undetected TP transmission throughout every community, with many of the infected unaware of what they had, what they were giving others, and what was yet to come.

References

1. Charles L. Ortleb, "No Syphilis Amnesty," *New York Native* (2/15/88): 6.
2. Henry H. Morton, M.D., "Genitourinary Diseases and Syphilis (C.V. Mosby Co.: 1918), 654.
3. Mandell, Douglas Jr., and Bennett, *Principles and Practices of Infectious Diseases* (John Wiley and Sons: 1979), 1825.
4. Henry H. Hazen, M.D., *Disease of the Skin* (C.V. Mosby, Co.: 1915), 273.
5. J.E. Moore, M.D., *Penicillin in Syphilis* (Charles C. Thomas, Publisher: 1946), 111.
6. Stokes, Beerman, and Ingraham, *Modern Clinical Syphilology*, 3rd ed. (W.B. Saunders Co.: 1944), 1251.
7. Wm. A. Hinton, M.D., *Syphilis and its Treatment* (The MacMillan Co.: 1936), 69–70.
8. *Ibid*, 81.
9. Stephen J. McPhee, M.D., "Secondary Syphilis: Uncommon Manifestations, a Common Disease," *The Western Journal of Medicine* (January 1984): 35; M.A. Conant, M.D. and B. Lane M.D., "Secondary Syphilis Misdiagnosed as Infectious Mononucleosis," *California Medicine* (December 1968): 462.
10. L.M. Drusin, M.D., et. al., "Infectious Syphilis Mimicking Neoplastic Disease," *Archives of Internal Medicine*, vol. 137 (February 1977): 156–160.
11. Thomas A. Chapel, M.D., "Physicians Recognition of the Signs and Symptoms of Secondary Syphilis," *Journal of the American Medical Association*, 7/17/81, vol. 246, no. 3, 250–251.
12. W.F. Felton, "Estimate of annual incidence of undiscovered syphilis," *British Journal of Venereal Diseases*, vol. 49 (1973): 249–255.
13. R.A. Smego, Jr., M.D., et. al, "Secondary Syphilis Masquerading as AIDS in a Young Gay Male," *North Carolina Medical Journal*, vol. 45, no. 4 (April 1984): 253–254.
14. J.A. Stroh, "The 'Great Imitator' Keeps Up with the Times," *Hospital Practice*, 11/15/86, 33.
15. Y.M. Felman, M.D., and J.A. Nikitas, M.A., "Syphilis Serology Today," Arch. Dermatol., vol. 116 (January 1980): 84–89.
16. P.F. Sparling, M.D., "Diagnosis and Treatment of Syphilis," *The New England Journal of Medicine*, vol. 284, no. 12 (3/25/71): 642.
17. S. William Becker, M.D., and Maximilian E. Obermayer, M.D., *Modern Dermatology and Syphilology* (J.B. Lippincott Co.: 1943), 881.
18. J. Lawton Smith, M.D., *Spirochetes in Late Seronegative Syphilis, Penicillin Not Withstanding* (Charles C. Thomas, Publisher: 1969), 64.

19. Mandell, et. al., *op. cit.*, 1831.
20. A.S. Sprangler, M.D., et. al, "Syphilis With a Negative Blood Test Reaction," *Journal of the American Medical Association*, vol. 189, no. 2 (7/13/64): 113.
21. Becker and Obermayer, *op. cit.*, 664.
22. *AABB Technical Manual*, 7th ed., American Association of Blood Banks (1977): 253; *Ibid*, 8th ed. (1981): 318.
23. L.M. Drusin, M.D., "Syphilis: Clinical Manifestations, Diagnosis, and Treatment," *Urologic Clinics of North America*, vol. 11, no. 1 (February 1984): 127.
24. Felman and Nikitas, *op. cit.*, 84–89.
25. R. Lindskov, et. al., "Acute HTLV-III Infection With Roseola-Like Rash," *Lancet*, (2/22/86): 447.
26. *Dorland's Illustrated Medical Dictionary*, 27th ed. (W.B. Saunders Co: 1988), "roseola" defined 1472.
27. J.A. Kolmer, M.D., *Serum Diagnosis by Compliment Fixation* (Lea and Febiger, Philadelphia: 1928), 485.

Chapter 8

Tragic Magic

Whatever measures may be taken by public authorities against the propagation of syphilis, it is always the medical profession who will take the chief part in the struggle.

—Professor Kaposi of Vienna[1]

Truly, the medical profession has played a critical role in making syphilis what it is today, and have wiped from our minds the horrors of generations past. No longer do people fear a lifetime of agony as consequence for a moment of bliss. We can rely upon our friendly physician to come to our rescue should we ever have reason to worry, for he knows what venereal evil lurks in the parts of men. Like a modern gunslinger on the side of good, today's doctor is ever ready with his fast six-shooter remedies: hypodermic, pill, drop, ointment, suppository, and catheter. He has what it takes to keep us clean. Or does he?

Twentieth-century medicine is founded upon the triad of patient, physician, and pharmacist, the goal being to bring your ailment under the gun of its specific magic bullet. The magic bullet concept arose from the work of Dr. Paul Ehrlich and his 1910 discovery of Salvarsan, the first effective treatment for syphilis. Ehrlich was searching for drugs which would kill disease causing organisms without harming patients. At the time of its discovery, Salvarsan was heralded as a tremendous therapeutic breakthrough for the treatment of TP infection. However, the concept of it being a magic bullet was not fulfilled, as it was found to be highly toxic and sometimes fatal. Yet, Ehrlich's achievement, though short of his intended goal, had a major influence upon modern medical therapeutics. Ever since then, like Ponce DeLeon and the fountain of youth, researchers have tried in vain to find the magic bullet for every ailment known to mankind. Unfortunately, as with Ehrlich, treatments which at first appeared to be ideal, sooner or later were discovered to have some drawback or downside. Though some good therapies have arisen from research, no magic bullets have been found, and in some cases, when the therapies are bad, there is only tragedy. Such is the story of syphilis.

Treponemal infections have for centuries been one of medicine's greatest challenges. While many attempts have been made to find means to kill the bacterium, most treatments have at best provided only symptomatic relief. However, even with symptomatic therapy the treponeme is left alive within its host, waiting for another opportunity to unleash its terror. Therefore, few approaches to TP have ever held the true potential of permanently curing syphilis, and there has never been a vaccine able to prevent infections.

Since the epidemic of the 1400s, there have been enough unsuccessful attempts at curing syphilis to fill a book. Though short of the curative goal, several of these remedies stand out as the best available treatments of their time. Unfortunately, while they did show evidence of being beneficial, they usually entailed some degree of risk to the patient. Exemplary of these were those therapies based on mercury, bismuth, iodides, and arsenic.[2] The mercurials are the oldest of the four, dating back to the 1490s, while bismuth treatments were begun in the 1920s. Like Salvarsan, a member of the arsenic family, these "cures" were often worse than the disease, with patients dying nearly as often as the treponemas. However, with the discovery of penicillin by Alexander Fleming in 1928, all of this would change.

Penicillin is known to have bacteriocidal abilities which make it the current drug of choice in the treatment of syphilis and many other bacterial infections. However, there are many forms of penicillin available for use against TP, and the choice of one over the other can make all the difference between success and failure. In addition, the amount used and duration of therapy are also important factors in determining success of therapy. The right combination of type, time, and amount can cure an illness, while misjudging any one of these may result in sub-therapeutic treatment or death.

Before the correct quantity and duration of application for any therapeutic drug can be determined, the drug's method of action must be understood. As was stated by Dr. J.E. Moore in 1946, "it is agreed that with all the penicillin-sensitive bacteria tested, the drug is active (whether by bacteriolysis, bacteriostasis, or direct bactericidal action) only against rapidly multiplying organisms in the stage of active growth . . . it is wholly or completely inactive against the same organisms in the resting phase." [3] The power of penicillin appears to lie in its ability to disrupt normal cell wall formation critical to successful reproduction.[4] In 1949, M.C. Cumberland and T.B. Turner calculated that after initial TP infection, the bacterium reproduced once every thirty hours.[5] However, the experiments upon which they based these calculations were only done for primary genital infections, without any research into infections of greater than three weeks duration. Also, only genital infections were investigated, while other areas of the body invaded by TP, like the central nervous system, were never studied. Many questions remain as to whether the rate of TP replication remains constant during infection, while the influence factors like intracellularity may have on reproduction is still unknown. Yet, incomplete as it is, the 1949 study has had tremendous impact. Many medical texts today still reference it as the definitive statement on TP reproduction,[6] from which they conclude "it can be implied that the most effective treatment would be to assume a sufficient blood level over a prolonged period of time . . . the most convenient way to achieve this goal is to treat with benzathine penicillin." [7] Here is where today's tragedy begins.

Benzathine penicillin G (BPG), one of the many forms of penicillin available to modern medicine, is the drug most often used against syphilis. This is due to the fact it maintains high antibiotic serum levels over long periods of time. Detectable levels of the drug have been found in the urine up to twelve weeks after a single 1.2 million unit intramuscular injection.[8] Thus, given Cumberland and Turner's assumption that all treponemas will replicate within thirty hours, BPG has been touted as the magic bullet for syphilis. Today, the American protocol for treatment of TP infection recommends the use of benzathine penicillin G, 2.4 million units, given intramuscularly at a single injection for patients without penicillin allergy.[9] Individuals showing advanced complications of syphilis may receive larger doses of BPG over longer time periods. This protocol has won immense popularity for BPG treatment of TP infection, as it is inexpensive and quick to administer, with no requirement for follow-up evaluation. However, a heavy price has been paid for the luxury of convenience. Due to its inherent biochemical limitations, it is impossible for BPG to cure treponemal infections.

It is usually assumed that the first notable sign of syphilis is a chancre appearing three weeks after initial infection. By this time, TP has spread throughout the body via the lymph and blood circulatory systems, achieving intracellularity in all parts of its host, including the central nervous system (CNS). By the time an infected individual is aware of their chancre (assuming one appears and is visible), visits their physician for blood tests samples, and the samples return confirming the presence of TP, additional weeks may pass before the administration of BPG begins. Hence, the treponeme has achieved intracellularity and invasion of the central nervous system long before benzathine penicillin enters the battle. Yet, while BPG can circulate for weeks within the blood, it cannot pass into the central nervous system. This is the fundamental tragedy in the use of this type of penicillin for treating syphilis.

As previously mentioned, Cumberland and Turner never studied BPG's inability to pass into the central nervous system. This portion of the body is protected by a special membrane known as the blood-brain barrier (BBB), which keeps the blood separate from the cerebrospinal fluid (CSF) which bathes the brain and spinal cord. This barrier prevents many substances from passing into the central nervous system. While TP can easily pass through the blood-brain barrier, benzathine penicillin G cannot and, therefore is not, able to kill the bacterium circulating in our cerebrospinal fluid. A 1976 article in the *Journal of the American Medical Association* summarized the problem as follows:[10]

> Wilner and Brody reported a failure rate of 39% in patients with neurosyphilis who were treated with penicillin in total doses of 3 to 30 million units parenter-

> ally. That is, in 39% of their patients, progressive neurologic signs developed following treatment. A failure rate of this magnitude supports our observation that many patients treated with benzathine penicillin G do not have spirocheticidal penicillin levels in their CSF.

This was echoed in a 1988 letter published in the same journal, which stated "the recommended drug for treatment of primary and secondary syphilis, penicillin G benzathine, does not reach treponemicidal levels in the CSF, so it is not unexpected that some 'adequately treated' patients who harbor spirochetes in their central nervous system develop neurosyphilis." [11] A European study published in 1987 also confirmed the 1976 study, noting "it has been reported that penicillin dosage regimens commonly used to treat late syphilis do not consistently reach treponemicidal concentrations in the CSF and are insufficient to treat syphilis when the CNS is affected." [12] How sad that in the pre-AIDS era when gays were finding the sexual freedom they had been denied for centuries, they were also being repeatedly infected with TP which their doctors repeatedly treated with Benzathine penicillin G. While the bacterium was removed from their peripheral blood system and their symptoms were abated, their central nervous systems underwent countless untreated invasions of TP. The 1960s and 1970s provided two decades of neurological inbreeding of this infection. It is little wonder that today we find ourselves in an AIDS epidemic so similar to the malignant syphilis epidemic of the 1400s.

Lamentably, few physicians ever do lumbar punctures for cerebrospinal fluid tests, even though CSF examination is essential to determine the central nervous system's involvement with syphilis. This lack of investigation has allowed doctors to claim successful cures, as corroborated by negative serum tests. Yet VDRL's and RPR's of the blood tell nothing about what is happening in the cerebrospinal fluid. Not only are the blind leading the blind, they are removing any hope of restoring sight and understanding of treponemal infection. Dr. W.A. Hinton recognized the importance of cerebrospinal fluid tests in 1936, long before the widespread use of penicillin, when he wrote:[13]

> In actual practice, even if guided by inferior blood tests, spinal fluid examinations are made on relatively few syphilitic patients, and for several reasons: (1) many

> physicians who must of necessity treat syphilitics have no ready facilities for the lumbar puncture; (2) its expense, if performed on every patient with syphilis, is greater than can reasonably be borne by most patients or most hospitals; (3) neurosyphilologists have not been able to convince many other physicians that, except in a small portion of cases, its value is commensurate with its inconvenience; (4) the attendant pain and other discomforts often make it difficult to obtain the patient's consent for the first lumbar puncture, and many times impossible to get permission for subsequent ones.

Nonetheless, Hinton urges that "a spinal fluid test is always indicated in those who have negative blood tests, signs of neurosyphilis, and no history of infection, because there are no other means of knowing whether the neurological symptoms are caused by syphilis or by some other disease." [14] His words still ring true over fifty years later, with AIDS patients continually showing neurological complications consistent with syphilis and physicians relying on inferior serum tests consistent with misdiagnosis.

The ineffectiveness of penicillin, though not completely recognized, has not been totally lost upon the Centers for Disease Control. Numerous cases of Benzathine penicillin G failure have been reported,[15] and a 1987 editorial in the *Journal of the American Medical Association*, by Dr. Mary E. Guinan of the CDC, included the following:[16]

> The treatment of syphilis is controversial. When comments were being solicited for updating the 1982 Centers for Disease Control Sexually Transmitted Diseases Treatment Guidelines, more questions were raised regarding syphilis treatment than any of the other 26 diseases or syndromes discussed. Unfortunately, not enough data are available to determine whether the recommended treatments are optimally effective or whether the efficacy of these regimens is stable. To evaluate treatment regimens, simplified strategies for determining cure of syphilis must be developed.

A 1979 medical text concurred with Guinan by complaining that "there has never been a well-controlled, carefully planned prospective study to determine the optimal dose or duration of [penicillin] therapy." [17] It is surprising, considering the intricacies involved in syphilitic infection, that Guinan would want to suggest simple strategies for further research. TP interferes with and produces many complex bio-chemical processes which require complex research to understand. It is the desire for easy answers which has led to the acceptance of the inferior BPG syphilis protocol, while maintaining our ignorance as a barrier between us and true curative treatment.

Antibiotics have been both a blessing and curse in disguise. While they have clearly demonstrated their importance in the fight against syphilis, not one of them has been conclusively shown to completely eradicate the organism from the human body. While Benzathine penicillin G may alleviate the external contagious manifestations of syphilis, it has never been able to cure the infection. Therefore, anyone previously treated with just the American syphilis protocol is still infected with live TP circulating inside their brain and spinal cord. A vast majority of the pre-AIDS gay community, which was epidemic with syphilis, falls into this category, including nearly all of those dead or dying of immunosuppression before the conscientious sex-habit changes of the mid-1980s.

While mainstream medicine stills adheres to the BPG protocol, and most syphilitics unwittingly undergo non-curative symptomatic treatment, others are looking at alternative antibiotics to use against TP. In 1985, the research results of Dr. C.W. Yim's work with doxycycline were published.[18] She and her associates administered two-hundred milligrams of the synthetic tetracycline orally twice a day for three weeks. They wrote, in a 1987 commentary that "the mean level of doxycycline in the cerebrospinal fluid of our patients was 26 percent of the simultaneous drug level in serum." [19] In comparison, a 1988 pharmaceutical manual notes that penicillin's "CSF levels usually do not exceed 5% of penicillin G's peak serum concentration." [20] While Yim declares "it should be emphasized that the spirocheticidal level of doxycycline in humans, both in cerebrospinal fluid and serum, remains to be determined," [21] its antisyphilitic properties and ability to pass through the blood-brain barrier, in concentrations five times those of BPG, make it an obvious choice for new research into improved treponemal therapies.

It is important to remember that while it cannot live up to the claims modern medicine has placed on it over the past thirty to forty years, Benzathine penicillin G may still play an important role in the ultimate eradication of TP. Some researchers, like Dr. Stephen Caiazza of New York City, are looking at the benefits of combining BPG and doxycycline treatments for AIDS patients. He believes syphilis is the fundamental infection of AIDS and has reported many positive results from his combined protocol (see Appendix B), while concurrently establishing important links between the two diseases. Meanwhile, several European researchers have demonstrated penicillin's ability to stop the spread of Kaposi's sarcoma,[22] a manifestation of both syphilis and AIDS. Studies like these clearly point out the need for new research into syphilitic diseases, their causes, and possible cures.

Today's epidemic is still in its infancy, but has already etched its place in history. Much of the AIDS story remains untold, with the most important part, the cure, still absent. Many tragedies have happened during the past decade, the most cruel of which may be yet to come. If, as the evidence suggests, AIDS is actually a malignant outburst of syphilis, a disease we have erroneously been led to believe is curable with BPG, then it is our blind resistance to seeing our mistakes which prevents us from ending this epidemic. The only way we will ever know the truth is to throw away the magic in favor of science.

References

1. Prof. Alfred Fournier, Paris, *The Treatment and Prophylaxis of Syphilis* (Rebman, Co., N.Y.: 1907), 461.
2. J.E. Moore, M.D., *The Modern Treatment of Syphilis*, 2nd ed. (Charles C. Thomas, Publisher: 1941), chapters 6, 8–10.
3. J.E. Moore, M.D., *Penicillin in Syphilis* (Charles C. Thomas, Publisher: 1946), 100.
4. *The United States Pharmacopoeial Dispensing Information*, 8th ed., The United States Pharmacopoeial Convention, Inc., vol. IB (1988): 1687.
5. M.C. Cumberland and T.B. Turner, "The Rate of Multiplication of Treponema Pallidum in Normal and Immune Rabbits," *American Journal of Syphilis, Gonorrhea, and Venereal Diseases*, vol. 33 (1949): 201.

6. Holmes, Mardh, Sparling, and Wiesner, *Sexually Transmitted Diseases* (McGraw-Hill Book Co.: 1984), 291.
7. Mandell, Douglas Jr., and Bennett, *Principles and Practices of Infectious Diseases* (John Wiley and Sons: 1979), 1833.
8. *American Hospital Formulary Service Drug Information*, The American Society of Hospital Pharmacists, Inc. (1988): 223–224.
9. J.E. Conte, Jr., M.D., and S.L. Barriere, Pharm. D., *The Manual of Antibiotics and Infectious Diseases*, 4th ed. (Lea and Febiger, Philadelphia: 1981), 224; A.L. Schroeter, et. al., "Treatment for Early Syphilis and Reactivity of Serologic Tests," *The Journal of the American Medical Association*, vol. 221, no. 5 (6/31/72): 471–476.
10. J.A. Mohr, M.D., et. al., "Neurosyphilis and Penicillin Levels in Cerebrospinal Fluid," *The Journal of the American Medical Association*, vol. 236, no. 19 (11/8/76): 2208.
11. M.L. Fernandez-Guerrero, M.D., et. al., "The Treatment of Neurosyphilis in Patients with HIV Infection," *The Journal of the American Medical Association*, vol. 259, no. 10 (3/11/88): 1495–1496.
12. van Eijk, et. al., "Effect of early and late syphilis on central nervous system: cerebrospinal fluid changes and neurological deficit," Genitourin Med, vol. 63 (1987): 81.
13. Wm. A. Hinton, M.D., *Syphilis and its Treatment* (The MacMillan Co.: 1936), 143–144.
14. *Ibid*, 144–145.
15. N.J. Fiumara, M.D., "Failure of Recommended Treatment for Secondary Syphilis," *The Journal of the American Medical Association*, vol. 256, no. 11 (9/19/86): 1443; D.M. Markovitz, M.D., et. al., "Failure of Recommended Treatment for Secondary Syphilis," *The Journal of the American Medical Association*, vol. 255, no. 13 (4/4/86): 1767– 1768; L.L. Bayne, M.D., et. al., "Acute Syphilitic Meningits: Its Occurrence After Clinical and Serological Cure of Secondary Syphilis With Penicillin G," *Arch. Neurol.*, vol. 43 (February 1986): 137–138; J. Jorgensen, et. al., "Neurosyphilis after treatment of latent syphilis with benzathine penicillin," *Genitourin Med*, vol 62 (1986): 129–131; E.C. Tramont, M.D., "Inadequate Treatment of Neurosyphilis with Penicillin," *The New England Journal of Medicine* (6/3/76): 1296; B.M. Greene, M.D., et. al., "Failure of Penicillin G Benzathine in the Treatment of Neurosyphilis," *Arch. Intern. Med.*, vol. 140 (August 1980): 1117–1118; E.C. Tramont, M.D., "Persistence of Treponema pallidum Following Penicillin G Therapy," *The Journal of the American Medical Association*, vol. 236, no. 19 (11/8/76): 2206– 2207; J.L. Smith, M.D., "Spirochetes in Late Seronegative Syphilis Despite Penicillin Therapy," *Medical Times*, vol. 96, no. 6 (June, 1968): 611–623.

16. M.E. Guinan, M.D., "Treatment of Primary and Secondary Syphilis: Defining Failure at Three- and Six-Month Follow-up," *The Journal of the American Medical Association*, vol. 257, no. 3 (1/16/87): 359.
17. Mandell, et. al., *op. cit.*.
18. C.W. Yim, M.D., et. al., "Penetration of oral doxycycline into the cerebrospinal fluid of patients with latent or neurosyphilis," Antimicrob Agents Chemother, vol. 28 (1985): 347–348.
19. C.W. Yim, M.D., et. al., Letter to the editor, *The New England Journal of Medicine*, vol. 317, no. 23 (12/3/87): 1474.
20. E.K. Kastrup, founding editor, *Facts and Comparisons Loose-leaf Drug Information Service* (J.B. Lippincott Co.: 1988), 382a.
21. C.W. Yim, M.D., et. al., *op. cit.*, 1987.
22. J. Fayolle, et. al., "La Penicilline Dans le Traitement de L'Angiosarcomatose de Kaposi," Lyon Medical, vol. 244, no. 17 (1980): 277–281; L. Pierini and D. Grinspan, "Resultados Obtenidos en el Tratamiento de la Sarcomatosis de Kaposi por la Penicilina," Revista Argentina de Dermatosifilologia, vol. 32, no. 1–2 (January–June 1948).

Chapter 9

World War Zero

Never neglect to inform your physician of your special antecedents. Tell him plainly, tell him ten times rather than once, that you have had syphilis.

—Alfred Fournier, 1907 [1]

War is one of our darkest acts. The overt destruction of life and its accomplishments had never been seen on a grander scale before the coming of mankind. Yet, while we can be the most monstrous of the animal kingdom, we can also be the most benevolent, expressing concern and compassion far beyond that of any other life-form. Though our kindness cannot always outshine our hate, it does remind us that we can live in peace, if we choose. While we may have perfected the art of cruelty on a global scale, we know by our love that we can change the way we act. It is this love which separates us from worlds where there is nothing but hostility.

Long before man picked up his first stone, hurling it malevolently in preparation for battles yet to come, a global conflict millions of years old was already raging. No other war has lasted longer, costs more lives, and is fought every day, by everyone, everywhere, than the one boiling inside of us: the immunological battle. Daily, we are besieged by thousands upon thousands of microorganisms, including bacteria, fungi, and viruses. They strike at our very existence, in what may be the ultimate test for survival. Standing between us and certain death is our immune system, fighting for us from cradle to grave. It is our largest and longest conflict in history, and the predecessor of all other world wars.

At the heart of AIDS lies our immune system and its ancient battle, which we are suddenly losing. The normal balance between health and disease, which our immune system safeguards, has been unexpectedly upset. Any explanation about the cause of AIDS needs to account for this weakening in our defenses. The syphilis theory, therefore, must be considered, as TP infection is known to cause immunosuppressive disease.

The 1980 text *Manual of Clinical Immunology* stated that "the immunological response to infection with T. pallidum is complex and poorly understood." [2] C.A. Mims, author of *The Pathogenesis of Infectious Diseases*, explained in 1982 that modern medicine was responsible for this as "patients who get syphilis are treated and immunologists have not had the opportunity to catch up with this disease." [3] While the present protocol for treating TP infection is not curative, it has hindered researchers in their investigation of the immune system's response to syphilis. Nevertheless, some progress has been made and, as noted in the 1988 medical text *Immunological Disorders*, "a number of authors have reported an impairment of lymphocyte function in patients with syphilis." [4]

Two key components of our immune system are T lymphocytes (T-cells) and B-lymphocytes (B-cells). When we are invaded by an antigen, foreign organisms such as bacteria or viruses, T- and B-cells play important roles in our defensive response. When T-cells, which are constantly circulating in our blood and lymph systems, come into contact with an antigen they react by producing other T-cells which have specific functions: effector, helper, suppressor, and memory T-cells. Effector T-cells emit substances called lymphokines which attract antigen-eating macrophages to the site of infection. The helper T-cells aid the B-cells in producing antibodies: molecular structures which attack the antigen. While the helper cells act as on-switches to facilitate B-cell activity, suppressor T-cells are the off-switch which inhibit further antibody production. Suppressor T-cells call off our defensive attack once the threatening antigen has been destroyed. Should the same antigen invade us again, our immune system will react more quickly the second time. Memory T-cells facilitate this faster reaction, known as an anamnestic response, which is the basis for immunization and vaccination. Vaccines produce these memory T-cells, setting the stage for the stronger anamnestic response, should we ever be infected by an organism we have previously been inoculated against.[5]

When T-cells react to antigens they produce other cells. Their reactions, therefore, are called cell-mediated or cellular immune responses. B-cells, on the other hand, produce antibody molecules, so their reactions are called humoral or antibody-mediated immune responses.[6] Normally, in a healthy individual's circulatory systems, there are almost twice as many helper T-cells as there are suppressor T-cells.[7] Hence, our immune system is prepared to "turn-on" and protect us against invading microorganisms. However, in AIDS there is an overall depletion in the number of T-cells, with the suppressors outnumbering the helper variety two-to-one. The weakened immune system is producing more "off" signals than "on" signals, and, therefore, is prevented from defending us from disease-causing antigens.

Syphilis has a profound impact upon the immune system and is unaffected by our B-cells' humoral responses. The 1978 medical text *Infectious Diseases* concluded "the most compelling evidence that humoral immunity does not protect the human host against syphilis is that these various antibodies are regularly demonstrated late in primary syphilis, yet do not appear to alter the progression to, or the manifestations of, secondary infection." [8] Though the B-cells reactivity is present shortly after infection, their antibodies do not protect us against treponemal disease. This ineffective B-cell response was noted in a 1977 article published in the medical journal *Infection and Immunity*, which demonstrated "selective impairment of T-cell function, whereas B-cell activity appears unchanged during the course of syphilitic infection." [9] It is not known what keeps the B-cells from making effective antibodies, but in the second edition of *The Pathogenesis of Infectious Diseases*, the author explained and speculated: [10]

> After infection with Treponema pallidum bacterial immobilizing antibodies are formed and there is an initial [cell mediated immune] response, as detected by marked lymphocyte transformation in vitro in the presence of treponemas. This initial response disappears as the bacteria multiply and spread through the body, and

> lymphocytes from patients with early secondary syphilis fail to respond in vitro to Treponema pallidum . . . It is not known why lymphocytes from patients with early secondary syphilis fail to respond to the infecting bacteria. Antigen-specific suppression is a possibility, or alternatively, T-cells are desensitized by circulating bacterial antigens.

Obviously, though we have yet to understand and explain it, syphilis is able to bypass our antibody-immune response in its progression of disease. This defiance of B-cell activity is likely to be closely related to syphilis' impact on our immune system's cell-mediated response.

While B-cells play a significant role in defending us against organisms like TP, "T lymphocytes are most important in defending against viruses, fungi, rickettsiae, and intracellular bacteria."[11] As previously noted, treponemas spread to all parts of the body, including the central nervous system, where they achieve intracellularity shortly after infection. Yet, while T-cells are crucial to effective defense against intracellular bacteria such as TP, they are not able to defend us against syphilis. The reason for this was summed up in a 1982 article of the *British Journal of Venereal Diseases*, when the authors stated:[12]

> In patients with syphilis, evidence has been found for a depression in cell mediated immunity, which involves cutaneous reactivity, low T-cell numbers, low in-vitro reactivity to Treponema pallidum, and immunosuppressive factors in serum. This study demonstrates that the total number of T lymphocytes are reduced in patients with early syphilis.

Long before the onset of AIDS, syphilis was known to cause both functional and population damage to T-cells. A decade before our modern plague began, medical journals were printing studies about TP's immunosuppressive abilities. In 1969, the British journal *Lancet* published an article titled "Reduced Lymphocyte Transformation due to a Plasma Factor in Patients with Active Syphilis," in which the authors summarized:[13]

> A factor is present in the plasma of patients with secondary syphilis which reduces the ability of normal lym-

> phocytes to be transformed. This factor could be a product of Treponema pallidum or an autoantibody. This impairment of lymphocyte function may be related to an impairment of cell-mediated immunity, which itself may be part of the mechanism of the development of the clinical manifestations of secondary syphilis.

A 1974 article in the same journal restated this theme as: [14]

> The immunological reaction in early syphilis is one that shows a partial inhibition of the cell-mediated response, which could account for the persistence of infectiousness and for the ease of demonstrating treponemas in the tissues. The incomplete immune response had been demonstrated by the results of the delayed hypersensitivity skin test and by the finding of depletion in the areas of lymph nodes closely related to T-cell activity and around the splenic follicular arterioles.

Though it was no secret to physicians before 1980, the importance of syphilitic immunosuppression would be completely overlooked once the AIDS era began. This blind-eye attitude towards TP's role in the reduction of T-cells and avoidance of B-cell humoral responses continues today, even as more papers appear testifying to the treponema's destruction of our immune system. While the 1970s continued to produce results which "support the hypothesis that human infection with T. pallidum is followed by a complex interaction between cellular and humoral immunity, the former being suppressed in primary and secondary stages," [15] and speculations that "the reduction in lymphocyte reactivity in secondary syphilis may therefore be related to the heavy antigenic overload that exists at that time," [16] it would be researchers of the 1980s who produced the most startling data.

While the United States has publicized itself as being at the forefront of AIDS research, it has done little to increase our understanding of syphilis. Therefore, it has been left up to Europeans like Jorgen R. Jensen, of the Department of Dermatology and Venereology at the University of Aarhus in Denmark, to pave the way for us. As many American physicians do not subscribe to medical journals from outside the United States, they are unaware of the work Jensen and his colleagues have been reporting. In a 1982 article published in the *British Journal of*

Venereal Diseases, titled "Alterations in T lymphocyte and T lymphocyte subpopulations in patients with syphilis," Jensen found that while all his syphilitic patients showed a decrease in the number of T-cells, suppressor and helper T-cells were affected differently. At the beginning of early TP infection the number of helper cells was reduced while the number of suppressor cells remained normal. Yet, as the early stages progressed, this trend was reversed. While their subjects were not known to be AIDS patients or suffering from multiple compounded treponemal infections, non-malignant syphilis was sufficient to cause these alterations. This led Jensen to theorize the possibility "that T. pallidum itself is directly toxic to T lymphocytes . . . [or] . . . T. pallidum may give an in-vivo stimulation, which in conjunction with immune complexes stimulates [suppressor] cells to release immunosuppressive factors." [17] That same year, and in the same journal, a second article by Jensen offered further evidence and affirmation that "the biological role of immune complexes in syphilis may be a direct 'shut off' signal to B-cells, a blocking of macrophages and their cooperation with lymphocytes, a stimulation of [T lymphocyte] cells to release immunosuppressive lymphokines, or a reduction in [natural killer] cell activity or both [*sic*]." [18] A third article published in 1984 by the *European Journal of Sexually Transmitted Diseases*, to which Jensen contributed, states that "during syphilis the number of T lymphocytes in blood is reduced with [*sic*] over 30%, independent of the stage of disease." [19] This latter study included patients with advanced, as well as early, TP infection, offering quantitative proof of the immunosuppression present in syphilitics.

It is unfortunate, given the devastation AIDS has caused in this country, that a known immunosuppressive disease like syphilis was not fully investigated by U.S. researchers. In actuality, most have never seriously considered the role TP infection may play in our epidemic. Dr. M.A. Fischl of the University of Miami School of Medicine, Division of General Medicine and Infectious Diseases, is a prime example of this. Fischl, who has conducted numerous studies on AIDS patients, was co-author of a 1983 article published in the *Annals of Internal Medicine*. "Opportunistic Infections and Kaposi's Sarcoma Among Haitians: Evidence of a New Acquired Immunodeficiency State" reported the results from a prospective study of eleven Haitians with AIDS pathology. Of the eleven, eight were positive on serum tests for treponemal infection. This led Fischl and her colleagues to conclude that "only serologic tests for syphilis and hepatitis B were significantly different from those of controls." [20] Yet, with syphilis clearly demonstrated in an overwhelming majority of this study group, the authors repeatedly contradicted themselves by stating "there was no evidence of an underlying immunosuppressive disease" [21]. Fischl and her associates ignored the fact that syphilis is a known immune system suppressor, even when seventy-three percent of their patients were infected with treponemas and immunosuppressed. In a 1988 television news interview, Fischl expressed her viewpoint concerning the use of syphilis therapies in AIDS, labeling the idea "absurd." [22] Quite to the contrary, given all the evidence, it is absurd that any researcher would eliminate TP from the list of organisms which may cause AIDS. Fortunately, not all scientists have been so rash.

As immune system dysfunction is crucial to the development of AIDS, immunostimulation offers an obvious starting point for treating patients. Salvatore Catapano, who holds one of only three U.S. patents granted for the treatment of AIDS, has turned to the typhoid vaccine for this purpose. The vaccine appears to induce increased immune system reactivity to all sorts of ailments other than typhoid, including AIDS. According to Catapano, who believes syphilis to be the fundamental infection responsible for AIDS, "it has been found that a complete immunization and remission of a person afflicted with AIDS, may be achieved by the parenteral administration with typhoid vaccine . . . with no observed toxicity." [23] In a recent article about Catapano, journalist Katie Leishman notes that "it is intriguing, however, that so many AIDS patients treated on the assumption that syphilis is their primary problem are well, while most of those who've received what is essentially antiviral treatment have died." [24]

The final answers to AIDS may be closer than we think. Perhaps we'll find the solution to be a combination of both vaccine and antibiotics. The greatest problem we face today, however, is getting more scientists involved in exploring syphilis' impact on our immune system and AIDS. While Jensen and his associates have provided crucial evidence of TP's immunosuppression, we lack the affirmative studies which account for the decades of multiple reinfections with TP and their subsequent inadequate therapeutic treatment which preceded this epidemic. While clearly leaders in their field, people like Salvatore Catapano and Dr. Stephen Caiazza represent only the beginning of overall research which needs to be done. Until then, our ignorance may continue to be the leading cause of death among people with AIDS.

References

1. Prof. Alfred Fournier, Paris, *The Treatment and Prophylaxis of Syphilis* (Rebman, Co., N.Y.: 1907), 303.
2. N.R. Rose and H. Friedman, *Manual of Clinical Immunology*, 2nd ed., The American Society for Microbiology (1980): 532.
3. C.A. Mims, *The Pathogenesis of Infectious Diseases*, 2nd ed., (Academic Press: 1982), 138.
4. M. Samter, M.D., *Immunological Disorders*, 4th ed. (Little, Brown and Co.: 1988), 824.
5. J.H. Cronenberger and J.C. Jennette, *Immunology: Basic Concepts, Diseases, and Laboratory Methods* (Appleton and Lange: 1988), 4.
6. *Ibid*, 8–11.
7. *Ibid*, 127.
8. M. Samter, M.D., *Infectious Diseases*, 3rd ed. (Little, Brown and Co.: 1978), vol. 2:642.
9. C.S. Pavia, et. al., "Selective Responses of Lymphocytes from Treponema Pallidum Infected Rabbits to Mitogens and Treponema Reiteri," *Infection and Immunity*, vol. 15 (1977): 420.
10. C.A. Mims, *op. cit.*, 138.
11. J.H. Cronenberger and J.C. Jennette, *op. cit.*, 12.
12. J.R. Jensen and E. From, "Alterations in T Lymphocytes and T Lymphocyte Subpopulations in Patients with Syphilis," *British Journal of Venereal Diseases*, vol. 58, (1982): 21.
13. G.M. Levene, et. al., "Reduced lymphocyte transformation due to a plasma factor with active syphilis," *The Lancet* (8/2/69): 246.
14. D.J.M. Wright and A.S. Grimble, "Why is the infectious stage of syphilis prolonged?," *British Journal of Venereal Diseases*, vol. 50 (1974): 48.
15. D.M. Musher, et. al., "Lymphocyte transformation in syphilis: an in vitro correlate of immune suppression in vivo?," *Infection and Immunity*, vol. 11, no. 6 (June 1975): 1261.
16. P.S. Friedman and J.L Turk, "A spectrum of lymphocyte responsiveness in human syphilis," *Clin. Exp. Immunol.*, vol. 21 (1975): 63.

17. J.R. Jensen and E. From, *op. cit.*.
18. J.R. Jensen, et. al., "Depression of natural killer cell activity by syphilitic serum and immune complexes," *British Journal of Venereal Diseases*, vol. 58 (1982): 300.
19. A.S. Jorgensen, et. al., "Immunosuppression in syphilis," *European Journal of Sexually Transmitted Diseases*, vol. 2 (1984): 8.
20. A.E. Pitchenik, et. al., "Opportunistic infections and Kaposi's Sarcoma among Haitians: evidence of a new acquired immunodeficiency state," *Annals of Internal Medicine*, vol. 98, no. 3 (March 1983): 282.
21. *Ibid*, 277.
22. During the week prior to Dr. Caiazza's March 13th, 1988 visit to Miami, a local network television station, channel 7 WSVN, broadcast a series of newscasts about Caiazza, one of which on March 11th included Dr. Fischl's reaction to his method of treating AIDS patients.
23. U.S. Patent No. 4,711,876.
24. Katie Leishman, "AIDS—Words From The Front," *Spin Magazine*, vol. 4, no. 8 (Nov. 1988): 47.

Chapter 10

Pandora's Other Box

For the tribes of men had previously lived on
earth
free and apart from evils, free from
burdensome labor
and from painful diseases, the bringers of
death to men.
In the power of these evils men rapidly pass
into old age.
But then [Pandora], raising the [box's] great
lid in her hands and
scattering its contents, devised anguishing
miseries for men.

—Hesiod (circa 700 B.C)[1]
Works and Days (90 – 95)

More than they produce answers, the previous chapters raise many questions, the most prominent of these being how could syphilis cause AIDS if all research is viral-oriented? While it is relatively easy to find evidence that TP is transmitted the same and produces the same manifestations as AIDS, that the American protocol for treating the disease doesn't work, and that syphilis is immunosuppressive, it is impossible to avoid the fact that no national study of syphilis is under way. This chapter will present a plausible and possible explanation of why, in the face of all this evidence, the syphilis theory is being ignored.

When Hesiod wrote his story of Pandora's box, in which the container was originally a jar, syphilis was undoubtedly among the evils released. Today, not to be outdone by the ancient Greek poet, we too have our own container full of misery and anguish far beyond that of our predecessor. Ours is the new Pandora's box: biological warfare (BW). With it we have surpassed Hesiod's messengers of death by creating means of contagious destruction.

Biological warfare is the willful use of microorganisms to inflict harm upon mankind. This may be done directly by using lethal agents which incapacitate or kill people, or indirectly by employing germs which attack agriculture or livestock. The debauchery of nature has become part of our modern military, with decades of research and development invested to produce a list of disease-causing weapons never before imagined. J.H. Rothschild, once Commanding General of the U.S. Army Chemical Corps Research and Development Command, wrote of this in his 1964 text *Tomorrow's Weapons*. His list of disease agents useful as biological weapons included anthrax, blastomycosis, botulism, brucellosis, cholera, coccidioidomycosis, crypttococcosis, dengue fever, bacillary dysentery, encephalitis, encephalomyelitis, glanders, influenza, melioidosis, bubonic plague, psittacosis, Q fever, Rift Valley fever, Rocky Mountain spotted fever, salmonella gastroenteritis, smallpox, tularemia, typhoid fever, typhus, and yellow fever.[2] Senator R.D. McCarthy, in his 1969 text *The Ultimate Folly*, added chikungunya fever to this list, while a 1984 article in *Science* magazine included Lassa fever, Ebola fever, Marburg disease, and hemorrhagic fevers.[3] Ultimately, any organism capable of producing disease is of interest to BW researchers.

Biological warfare has a long history in United States military affairs, going back as far as the American Civil War. With the goal of battle being to defeat the enemy with minimal expenditure of energy and lives, BW becomes the ideal weapon. Confederate General J.E. Johnston used a BW strategy in the Yorktown Peninsula Campaign of 1862, in which his troops occupied the high terrain above the Chickahominy lowlands. With his superior position, Johnston was able to pin down the opposing Union forces of General G.B. McClellan in the low lying, disease-infested swamp areas. With little effort on the part of the Confederates, nearly a regiment per day of Union soldiers were lost to disease. When Johnston was criticized for inactivity against his foe, he aptly replied, "I am fighting, sir, every day! Is it nothing that I compel the enemy to inhabit the swamps, like frogs, and lessen their strength every hour, without firing a shot?" [4]

The Civil War may well have been the birthplace of American biological warfare. Since then, it has been refined into the deadliest form of weaponry in existence, with a 1972 *Bulletin of the Atomic Scientists* explaining that "biological agents can theoretically inflict more casualties per weight than chemical, conventional, or nuclear weapons." [5] The superiority of BW over other modes of warfare was well known long before 1972, as a 1963 *Newsweek* article reported the following: [6]

> From a purely military standpoint, it is entirely possible—and entirely plausible—that biological weapons may someday be employed. For one thing, the area of their effectiveness far outstrips that of nuclear weapons: 450 pounds of a concentrated agent would blanket 34,000 square miles; a 20 megaton bomb will cause severe burns within 2,800 square miles . . . In many ways bacteria are the ultimate weapons.

The superiority of BW spawned increasing interest in and evolution of its technology. Research and development moved so quickly, that by 1986 the former deputy assistant secretary of defense for negotiations policy, Douglas Feith, reportedly stated: [7]

> BW can be designed to be effective across the spectrum of combat, including special operations and engagements at the tactical level, and that agents can now be developed that can neither be detected nor defended against . . . the prevailing judgement of years ago that BW is not a militarily significant weapon is now quite unsubstantiated.

As a group, scientists were well aware of BW's devastating potential long before most others. Unlike militarists who courted it for reasons of power, they have seen BW for the horror it really is. In 1964, the Federation of American Scientists released a statement condemning further research and development of BW technology.[8] In 1966, a group of twenty-two American scientists, including seven Nobel Laureates, sent a letter to President Johnson pleading with him to stop the development and use of biological weapons.[9] Unfortunately, as with other modes of devastating warfare, their discoveries were valued while their words of caution were ignored. This is most evident in federal spending on BW research, which has totalled well over a quarter of a billion dollars in this decade alone. While it did reach a low of fifteen million dollars allocated in 1981, by 1987 the yearly allocation was well over seventy million dollars.[10]

Genetic engineering has been one of the main reasons for the increased spending for biological warfare research, which a 1975 *Science* magazine article explained as follows: [11]

> The army's biological warfare scientist at Fort Detrick, Maryland, labored for many years to enhance the unpleasantness of microorganisms noxious to man. They are said to have had little success by the time that offensive biological warfare was renounced by President Nixon in November, 1969. The newly developed art of creating recombinant DNA molecules with restriction enzymes affords an obvious means of succeeding where Fort Detrick failed. The technique renders conceivable a Frankensteinian microbiology in which it would be possible, for example, to equip the human gut commensal Escherichia coli with genes for botulinum toxin.

It is hard to imagine anyone wanting to change organisms necessary for our survival into life threatening germs. Yet, long before this article was published, the U.S. Department of Defense was looking well beyond what can cause a disease, to focus on what keeps us safe from disease: our immune system. In 1969, a department spokesman stated the following: [12]

> Within the next five to ten years, it would probably be possible to make a new infective micro-organism which could differ in certain important respects from any known disease-causing organisms. Most important of these is that it might be refractory to the immunological and therapeutic processes upon which we depend to maintain our relative freedom from infectious diseases.

This quote, used by Robert Harris and Jeremy Paxman in their 1982 text *A Higher Form of Killing*, appears to predict the coming AIDS epidemic. Based upon this and other information, many authors have reasoned that AIDS is the direct result of a BW project gone mad. Dr. Alan Cantwell, Jr., author of *AIDS and the Doctors of Death*, explains how HIV could have been bioengineered from parts of visna virus and bovine leukemia virus, and then spread to unsuspecting victims via contaminated hepatitis-B vaccine.[13] Given there is little doubt our military had the technological know-how to do such a thing, and the strong correlation between the timing of the hepatitis vaccinations and the appearance of AIDS in populations given the vaccines, Cantwell presents a noteworthy scenario. Unfortunately, conclusive evidence supporting his claim is hard to find. The BW program has been, and still is, shrouded in a cloak of secrecy. It is difficult for any but those directly involved in biological warfare research to know what has happened, and what is currently being done. Even though, in support of Cantwell's thesis, enough was known in 1982 for Harris and Paxman to state: [14]

> The possibility that such a 'super germ' may have been successfully produced in a laboratory somewhere in the world in the years since that assessment was made is one which should not be too readily cast aside (6) . . . This is not an entirely academic speculation. In 1968 Porton Down [England] and Fort Detrick collaborated in the successful transfer of genes between different strains of plague bacillus.

Secrecy is probably the key word when it comes to BW research. While nuclear warfare and star wars technology are bantered about in the press and other news media, biological warfare is seldom heard of or seen. Much of this is due to a 1969 decision by President Richard Nixon, who shortly after taking office ordered a review of the biological warfare program then in progress. He discovered that millions of dollars were being thrown into a program which had neither defined goals nor procedures.[15] In addition, hundreds of experiments were done which threatened the lives of countless Americans. One of these was code-named Operation Seaspray, in which for six days during 1950 the U.S. Navy sprayed the bacterial agent Serratia Marcesens on San Francisco from ships steaming up and down the harbor.[16] An estimated 800,000 residents were exposed to the bacteria, which is now known to cause "every conceivable kind of infection, including those of the respiratory tract (lung abscess, bronchiectasis, pneumonia, and empyema) and urinary tract, meningitis, otitis media, peritonitis, endocarditis, infections of the musculoskeletal system (septic arthritis and osteomyelitis), wounds . . . lymphadenitis, and infections of the skin." [17] Though the Department of Defense claims it did not know the bacteria was harmful, a 1982 article in *The Nation* reports that "as far back as 1952 a secret memorandum prepared by the army revealed its concern that these bacteria were causing disease." [18] One man is known to have died from Serratia Marcesans pneumonia shortly after the San Francisco experiment, at a hospital which also reported ten other concurrent cases of the then rare pneumonia.[19]

Dozens of other places were sprayed by the U.S. military, including the New York City subway system, Minneapolis, parts of Alaska, Hawaii, the Pennsylvania Turnpike, Washington's National Airport, and Key West, Florida.[20] All in all, there were over two hundred of these open air tests done between 1949 and 1969. By all standards they were irresponsible and horrific experiments with incalculable risks. More disturbing is the fact that the San Francisco test was a repeat of earlier experiments done by the Nazis on British subway systems in the 1930s.[21] Nixon had every right to be disturbed by the results of his 1969 investigation.

In response to what he found, President Nixon changed the course of American BW policy by starting negotiations on an international treaty banning further offensive BW research. He also rededicated the army's biological warfare laboratories at Fort Detrick, Maryland, to become part of the National Institutes of Health's cancer research labs.[22] However, the Army was to maintain a small portion of the original facilities, which was renamed the United States Army Medical Research Institute of Infectious Diseases (USAMRIID), also known as Walter Reed Army Institute of Research.[23] In 1972, USAMRIID's commanding officer, Col. Dan Crozier, M.D., stated their primary task was "developing workable medical defenses against biological agents." [24] As restated in a 1984–85 issue of *Foreign Policy*, "today the U.S. biological defense research program, administered by the army, focuses on developing vaccines." [25] Here is where the story of AIDS may begin.

Biological warfare, as previously mentioned, is the most destructive form of conceivable warfare. Unfortunately, it is also one of the cheapest. With the help of recombinant DNA technology, the United States has been at the forefront of developing a deadly form of weaponry which almost any country can afford. Whereas it costs billions of dollars to create a nuclear weapons arsenal, a willing aggressor could synthesize previously unknown BW agents for mere millions. What is worse, once released, these weapons could not only produce more devastation than nuclear devices, but there would be no way to effectively detect them or defend against them. We have literally given our enemies the technology and know-how to destroy us. The only hope we have against such attacks is to learn how to develop quick and reliable vaccines. At the heart of this lay viruses, the smallest biological units containing life-giving, or taking, DNA.

The science of vaccines has been very slow and produced few results. We cannot even vaccinate ourselves against some of the most common ailments, like the cold. Even when a vaccine is developed, as in the case of influenza, the causative organism rapidly changes into a form unaffected by the vaccinations, yet just as threatening to our health. The Department of Defense is under considerable pressure to learn all it can of the science of vaccines before someone decides to test our ability to withstand a BW attack. To do this requires a large study population with whom to experiment. Unfortunately, due to public abhorrence of BW, the Pentagon has resorted to and been caught using devious and deceptive means to get budget allocations for BW projects.[26] This is where AIDS comes in.

Back in the 1960s, there was enough medical and scientific literature showing syphilis was able to cause almost every ailment known to mankind. In addition, there was evidence that it impaired the immune system, the protocol for treating syphilis was not curative, and TP would cause a myriad of bizarre manifestations if allowed to become malignant. With the sexual revolution of the sixties and seventies well underway, the disease was known to be epidemic in the gay community, which was a large part of the clientele of many inner-city health clinics. By discontinuing follow-up tracking of gay men with syphilis, as was done in New York City during the early 1970s,[27] the disease was allowed to spread unchecked and avoid effective treatment. The same thing was happening in Africa which has a history of epidemic treponemal infections and poor health controls. Communities, unwittingly being developed as study populations, were allowed to interbreed syphilitic infections in hopes of the malignant explosion which occurred shortly before 1980: AIDS. With this came millions of dollars to finance viral research, and thousands of guinea pigs with whom to experiment, all under the guise of public health. Aided by the general ignorance of professional and lay people alike concerning the nature of malignant syphilis, it was not hard to convince everyone that a virus was the cause of this new epidemic.

Our bodies play continual hosts to hundreds of different viruses, which under normal circumstances cause us no harm. Given the bizarre pathology manifested by malignant syphilis, it would only be a matter of time, which turned out to be four years (1979 to 1983), before some virus—any virus—would be found which could be declared the culprit. In those early years, there was no one around with enough experience, credentials, or financing to challenge the National Institutes of Health's viral theorists, who bought into the ploy hook, line, and sinker. For decades, the NIH had been unsuccessfully attempting to prove virus' were the cause of cancer, and now they were being offered millions to pursue their dying dream.[28] Though the virus itself was merely a front and not the fundamental AIDS disease, it produced funding for badly needed viral research: research which could save the NIH's reputation, and be of immense value to our nation's defense. It is a global con game which nets millions of dollars to finance research and thousands of willing guinea pigs with whom to experiment. It is also genocide.

While it is unwise to yell "the sky is falling," it is insane not to recognize when it has already fallen. Though the above scenario suffers the same lack of conclusive documentation as did Cantwell's, the overwhelming volume of circumstantial supporting evidence is undeniable. In addition, the following points should be considered:

1) Campaigns of disinformation about BW-related activities have previously occurred, as was the case with Operation Blue Sky, a 1950 government propaganda cam-

paign to convince the American public biological warfare is humane.[29]

2) With recombinant DNA technology, the U.S. Department of Defense has the technological ability to create new and lethal life-forms.
3) Biological weapons are cheaper and more devastating than nuclear weapons.
4) The United States has no means of effectively detecting or defending itself against a biological attack.
5) Our government spends more and more each year on defensive (vaccine) biological research.
6) The Department of Defense, in 1969, predicted that by 1970 there would be a microorganism which could destroy our immune system.
7) The Department of Defense has secretly and willfully exposed millions of Americans to disease-causing biological agents. In 1977 an army spokesman reportedly told a Senate hearing that these types of tests "might be resumed whenever the army felt a need." [30]
8) For forty years spanning the 1930s into the 1970s, the U.S. Public Health Service oversaw the Tuskegee syphilis experiment, in which over 400 black men were denied treatment for their syphilitic infections. Many of them died from syphilis, as a direct result of that experiment." [31]
9) Ten years of U.S. governmental AIDS research has produced antiviral drugs which do not cure patients. Even when properly administered, these drugs are highly toxic.[32]
10) The United States has a long history of deadly bigotry and abuse concerning those most affected by AIDS: blacks and homosexuals.

With a history of bigotry and abuse towards minorities deemed socially undesirable in this country, our government has both the motives, means, and experience in conducting covert actions against its own people. It cost our government little to mistreat and allow syphilis to become malignant, and it has produced an invaluable resource of subjects for human experimentation. Through the silence of syphilis, the guinea pigs of today's research may save us from biological destruction.

References

1. R.M. Frazer, *The Poems of Hesiod* (University of Oklahoma Press: 1983), 99.
2. J.H. Rothschild, *Tomorrow's Weapons* (McGraw-Hill: 1964), 198–205.
3. R.D. McCarthy, M.C., *The Ultimate Folly* (Knopf: 1969), 68–73; R.J. Smith, "New Army Biowarfare Lab Raises Concern," Science, *vol. 226 (12/7/84): 1176.*
4. Dr. P.E. Steiner, *Disease in the Civil War: Natural Biological Warfare in 1861–1865* (Charles C. Thomas, Publisher: 1968), 138–139.
5. P.A. Karber, "The Nixon Policy on CBW," *Bulletin of the Atomic Scientists*, vol. 28 (January 1972): 22.
6. "The Ultimate Weapon?" *Newsweek*, vol. 61 (3/4/63): 56.
7. S. Wright, "New Designs for Biological Weapons, *Bulletin of the Atomic Scientists*, vol. 43 (January–February 1987): 44.
8. "FAS Statement on Biological and Chemical Warfare," *Bulletin of the Atomic Scientists*, vol. 20 (October 1964): 46–47.
9. "Scientists Speak Out on CB Weapons," *Bulletin of the Atomic Scientists*, vol. 22 (November 1966): 39–40.
10. S. Shulman, "Funding for Biological Weapons Research Grows Amidst Controversy," *BioScience*, vol. 37, no. 6 (June, 1987): 372.
11. N.W., "Arms Control Report Card—Nuclear Treaty: Fatal Flaw . . . Biological Warfare: Unexpectedly Good," *Science*, vol. 189 (9/5/75): 772–773.
12. R. Harris and J. Paxman, *A Higher Form of Killing: the Secret Story of Chemical and Biological Warfare* (Hill and Wang, Publisher: 1982), 241.
13. Dr. A. Cantwell, Jr., *AIDS and the Doctors of Death: an Inquiry into the Origin of the AIDS Epidemic* (Aries Rising Press: 1988).
14. R. Harris and J. Paxman, *op. cit.*, 241, 266.
15. Statement by President Nixon released 11/25/69, "Chemical and Biological Defense Policies and Programs," Department of State Bulletin (12/15/69): 541.
16. L.A. Cole, "The Army's Secret Germ War Testing," *The Nation* (10/23/82): 397; N.C., "How the U.S. Used its Citizens as Guinea Pigs," *Saturday Review*, vol. 6 (11/10/79): 10.
17. V.L. Yu, M.D., "Serratia Marcesens: Historical Perspective and Clinical Review," *The New England Journal of Medicine*, vol. 300, no. 16 (4/19/79): 887.
18. L.A. Cole, *op. cit.*.
19. R.P. Wheat, M.D., et. al., "Infection due to Chromobacteria: Report of Eleven Cases," *A.M.A. Archives of Internal Medicine*, vol. 88 (October 1951): 461–466.

20. B. Chisholm, "Biological Warfare: Demand for Answers," *Bulletin of the Atomic Scientists*, vol. 15 (May 1959): 209–211; E.R., "The BW Threat," *Bulletin of the Atomic Scientists*, vol. 16 (June 1960): 244–246; S.M. Hersh, "Germs and Gas as Weapons," *The New Republic*, vol. 160 (6/7/69): 13–16; J. Hay, "The Summer and Smoke of '53," *Maclean's*, vol. 93 (5/26/80): 21–22; C. Piller, "DNA—Key to Biological Warfare?" *The Nation*, vol. 237 (12/10/83): 585, 597–601; L.A. Cole, "Operation Bacterium," *The Washington Monthly*, vol. 17 (July–August 1985): 38–45.
21. Wickham Steed, "Aerial Warfare: Secret German Plans," *The Nineteenth Century and After* (July 1934), 1–15; *The National Medical Dictionary* (Lea Brothers and Co.: 1890), see the definition for Micrococcus Prodigiosus, 153; *Blakiston's Gould Medical Dictionary*, 4th ed. (McGraw-Hill Book Co.: 1979), see the definition for Bacillus Prodigiosus, 148.
22. A. Kanegis and L. Richards, "The Budget Gives the Game Away," *The Nation*, vol. 213 (10/11/71): 337–340; M.S. Meselson, "Chemical and Biological Weapons," *Scientific American*, vol. 222, no. 5 (May 1970): 15–25.
23. N. Wade, "Biological Warfare Fears May Impede Last Goal of Smallpox Eradicators," *Science*, vol. 201 (7/28/78): 329 – 330.
24. R.A. Fineberg, "No More Chemical/Biological War?," *The New Republic*, vol. 167 (12/2/72): 17.
25. J.B. Tucker, "Gene Wars," *Foreign Policy* (Winter, 1984/1985): 69.
26. R.J. Smith, "New Army Biowarfare Lab Raises Concerns," *Science*, vol. 226 (12/7/84): 1176–1178.
27. J.E. D'Eramo, Ph.D., "Targeted for Negligence: Why I Resigned From the New York City Health Department," *Christopher Street*, issue 122 (May 1988): 19.
28. Dr. A. Cantwell, Jr., *op. cit.*.
29. R. Clarke, *The Silent Weapons* (David McKay Co., Inc.: 1968), 26.
30. L.A. Cole, "Yellow Rain or Yellow Journalism," *Bulletin of the Atomic Scientists*, vol. 40 (August–September 1984): 38.
31. J.H. Jones, *Bad Blood: The Tuskegee Syphilis Experiment* (The Free Press: 1981).
32. D.D. Richman, M.D., et. al., "The Toxicity of Azidothymidine (AZT) in the Treatment of Patients with AIDS and AIDS-Related Complex," *The New England Journal of Medicine* (7/23/87): 192–197.

Chapter 11

Commencement

I say, if it's love, the Lord won't mind.
There's enough hate in the world.
—Mrs. Sapphire Hall, Harlem, 1940[1]

AIDS continues to kill more Americans every day. As of October 24th, 1988, the CDC reported there were over 43,000 known deaths from the disease.[2] In the two month period between the writing of the first chapter of this book and this final chapter, nearly 3,000 AIDS patients have died: approximately fifty people each and every day, one every half hour. During this time, the CDC made a startling announcement. In the October seventh issue of their publication *Morbidity and Mortality Weekly Report*, they stated the following: [3]

> The frequency of unusual clinical and laboratory manifestations of syphilis in patients co-infected with HIV is unknown . . . Persons with HIV infection acquired through sexual contact or intravenous (IV) drug abuse should be tested for syphilis . . . When clinical findings suggest syphilis is present, but serological test are negative, other tests should be used . . . Recommended treatment schedules for neurosyphilis have included benzathine penicillin, although treatment with benzathine penicillin in currently recommended dosages does not achieve treponemicidal levels in the cerebrospinal fluid of most patients with syphilis . . . Benzathine penicillin regimens should not be used to treat either asymp-

> tomatic or symptomatic neurosyphilis in HIV-infected patients.

It is encouraging to see the CDC finally beginning to recognize the importance of syphilis in AIDS. Though they have yet to study TP as the fundamental immunosuppressive organism, this is a significant move towards meaningful research in this area.

This book has presented an introduction to many of the complex issues and contradictions surrounding syphilis and the AIDS epidemic. Some people simply will not care, most of them probably never considering to read this text. Others will view it as total hogwash, many of them never finishing it. Its absurdity will be reinforced by our government's non-response to both syphilis as AIDS, and AIDS in general. People having either of these viewpoints probably have not had to personally deal with the horror of AIDS. Not being directly affected, they would feel much as did James J. Kilpatrick when, in June of 1988, he wrote his Universal Press Syndicated column titled "AIDS panic: What's the big deal?," in which he says: [4]

> But it is also entirely appropriate, as the commission recommended, that the states make it a crime for persons knowingly to engage in sexual conduct likely to transmit the AIDS virus. I would treat AIDS for what it is: a disease that mortally afflicts a tiny fraction of the population whose willful behavior results in the infection . . . Let us apportion our tears, and our tax dollars, with some sense of proportion.

I seriously doubt Mr. Kilpatrick meant to apply his standards to heterosexuals. While most gays have made appropriate behavior changes to protect themselves from the epidemic, an illusion of immunity still seems prevalent among heterosexuals. It is not surprising that as the rate of new infections for gays declines, it is steadily increasing for heterosexuals. Overall, in the U.S. and worldwide, AIDS is still spreading at a geometric rate.

A third way to react to this book is to consider it conclusive evidence which validates the syphilis theory beyond a shadow of a doubt. While as an author it may be pleasing to find somebody in agreement with me, it would be a disappointment to have someone hold this text up as the gospel of AIDS.

Anyone believing this text has all the answers has made the same mistakes of those with either of the two previous reactions. The goal of this text has not been to say agree with me or you are wrong. The goal of this text is to make others aware that there are many serious questions concerning syphilis and AIDS which have yet to be addressed by those we trust to safeguard our health. In the words of Dr. Stephen Caiazza "I do not pretend to have all the answers . . . I may not have any of the answers, but I do have a lot of questions." [5]

It is my hope that you, the reader, will also come away from this book with this kind of reaction: a lot of questions. If you have ever had syphilis or AIDS, if you've known someone who has ever had syphilis or AIDS, or if you're just concerned about the AIDS epidemic, please don't stop asking questions every day and every way you can about this dreadful disease. Understand that every individual makes a difference in this issue, and that you cannot wait for anyone else before you get involved. In 1988, President Ronald Reagan clearly demonstrated this when he declared October to be National AIDS Awareness and Prevention Month. As has been typical of our government's criminal neglect of this issue, the proclamation to increase "awareness of the dread disease was signed by President Reagan on Oct. 28 and not made public until the month had ended." [6] Especially if you are gay, now more than ever, you must stand up for what is right, because nobody else is going to do it for you.

As a gay American, I have written this book with a clear commitment to help stop this epidemic. It is a tragedy that our country is currently dominated by homophobic policies which clearly inhibit progress towards a solution to AIDS. I feel anger that I and men and women like me are being repressed by a minority of narrowminded bigots. Yet, I feel a similar anger toward my community that it allows these bigots to manipulate the American system to take advantage of and repress us. Few of us know our own strength, for if we did we would come out and stand up for our rights as Americans. Until we do that, we cannot expect anyone else to give us the respect or help which we will not give ourselves.

A close friend of mine, after hearing what I was writing, criticized me for wanting to only look at the bad side of our country. He was upset with me for writing something that spoke so unfavorably of our nation, which I obviously did not appreciate. He was wrong. I love America and am not willing to turn my back when I see it doing wrong. I think too highly of it to expect anything but the best from it. Though as an individual I cannot solve the problems of this world, or even one country, I am doing my part so that one day America may be a little closer to the ideal it currently falls short of. Until then, we who do not participate in change are just as responsible for our woes as those who impose injustice upon us. It is time to stand up and be counted, to make a difference, and to live.

References

1. Gordon Merrick, *The Lord Won't Mind* (Avon Books: 1970).
2. The CDC number of known deaths from AIDS was 43,027 as of October 24, 1988. This figure was obtained from the National AIDS Hotline (1-800-342-2437), which receives monthly updates from the CDC.
3. "Recommendations for Diagnosing and Treating Syphilis in HIV-Infected Patients," *Morbidity and Mortality Weekly Report*, vol. 37, no. 39 (10/7/88): 600–608.
4. James J. Kilpatrick, "AIDS panic: What's the big deal?," *The Miami Herald* (6/9/88): 21A.
5. Dr. Stephen Caiazza, see Appendix B.
6. "White House declares AIDS Awareness Month—for October," *The Miami Herald* (11/2/88): 9A.

Chapter 12

Afterword

But what we also think is that, in spite of all our efforts, in spite of the long and active treatment, it is not impossible that this patient may be liable, in the more or less remote future, to some syphilitic or parasyphilitic manifestation. For unfortunately, there is no sign which allows us, in the case of syphilis, to affirm a cure.

Alfred Fournier, 1907 [1]

I completed the original text of this book in October 1988, and then spent more than a year writing over three hundred publishers in an attempt to make this information available to others.

As part of the publication process, I was asked to update the manuscript with an afterword. A lot has happened since I finished the original text of the book, though, unfortunately, there is little good news to share at this time. The number of known deaths, as reported to and compiled by the CDC has jumped from 43,027 in October 1988 to 68,441 by November 1989.[2] This forty percent increase of 25,414 more known deaths represents one AIDS fatality every 22½ minutes. AIDS patients are dying at a rate seven and a half minutes faster than at this same time last year (see chapter 11). The clock is ticking, time is running out, and we are losing.

The profoundness of our situation became strikingly clear to me during my first proofreading of the publisher's edition of this text. While reviewing the introduction, which describes how I originally became involved in this issue, I stopped and began to cry. The clarity of purpose, to which I was and still am dedicated, stood in stark contrast to the implications of what this book is stating: there is enough current medical and scientific literature in publication to support and justify national and international research which will determine the exact relationship between syphilis and AIDS—research which is not being done.

Though the research is absent, this does not mean there is nobody out there attempting to educate the public and our government about this subject. In the past year, Joan McKenna's article "Syphilis: The Legacy of War" was published in the April 1989 issue of *MINERVA: A Quarterly on Women in the Military*,[3] and Dr. Stephen Caiazza's book *AIDS: One Doctor's Personal Struggle* was also released.[4] Finally, Professor Peter H. Duesberg's article "Human Immunodeficiency Virus and Acquired Immunodeficiency Syndrome: Correlation but not causation," was printed in the February 1989 issue of the *Proceedings of the National Academy of Sciences*.[5] I was struck by the title of Professor Duesberg's article, and its relationship to that of a 1984 article titled "Correlation Between Exposure to Human T-Cell Leukemia-Lymphoma Virus-III and the Development of AIDS." It was in the earlier article that Dr. Robert Gallo and his associates first declared: [6]

> In particular, a high correlation between exposure to HTLV-III, detected by antibodies to HTLV-III in patient sera, and the development of AIDS was found. Based upon these observations, we conclude that HTLV-III is the primary cause of AIDS.

This declaration of causation based upon correlation harps back to the nineteenth century theory of spontaneous generation, also known as abiogenesis.[7] This antiquated concept stated that living matter could be derived from dead matter, and was founded upon observations such as the high correlation of flies which appeared to be spontaneously born from decaying meat. The famous Koch postulates of the nineteenth century were formulated in an attempt to prevent correlation from being mistaken as causation: postulates which the HIV theorist of today have yet to satisfy in terms of the disease AIDS.[8] How frightening this all becomes when one realizes that Gallo's high correlation was really present in only forty percent of the AIDS symptomatic subjects in his study. Unbelievably, a year earlier, Dr. M.A. Fischl and her associates reported finding seventy-three percent of their AIDS symptomatic subjects infected by Treponema pallidum (TP).[9] Yet, like flies to feces, we have spent the last ten years in the spontaneous misconception that HIV is the undeniable and only causative agent in AIDS.

We are living in a time of unprecedented spirochaetal adaptive radiation: the subtle and constant changes through which an organism evolves due to environmental influences.[10] In particular, TP, the causative agent of syphilis, is expanding and expressing itself into heretofore unknown areas. This bacterium is identical to the organisms which cause many other spirochaetal diseases, including endemic syphilis (also known as bejel), yaws, and pinta.[11] I must re-stress the word identical, because, though each disease has a different name, though each disease has a somewhat different pathology, and though the agent responsible for each disease has been given a unique title, if the causative agents for each of these diseases were simultaneously placed before a scientist for identification, there is no known chemical or physical means by which that scientist may tell any of them apart solely by the samples of these bacterium. The causative agent of Lyme disease, Borrelia burgdorferi, another spirochete, is so closely related to TP, both morphologically and pathologically, that it would appear to be a sub-strain of Treponema pallidum which has chosen an animal vector (Ixodes tick) for transmission rather than the traditional sexual mode.[12] I contend that what we are really witnessing is not the work of a new organism, but the same organism and its radiated offspring expressing themselves under the influence of varying environmental factors. In the case of AIDS, concurrent factors which include the non-curative syphilis therapy protocols combined with the sexual and drug revolutions of the 1960s and 1970s provided the opportunity for TP to express itself in its most devastating form known: malignant syphilis.

So, perhaps we have come full circle and have progressed no further than our ancestors of the 1400s. We repeat history because we refuse to remember it. Yet, how the community affected the most by this plague, the gay community, my community, can be, in general, so ignorant about the syphilis/ AIDS issue is beyond me. Legally, we are, as we have been for centuries, second-class citizens in the United States. Yet, we make up the majority of those dead and dying from AIDS, and we have willfully demanded and participated in experimentation based upon viral theories of AIDS without questioning the motives and morals of those we have entrusted to conduct these experiments. How can we passively place our future in the hands of a government which on local and national levels has done little other than express its contempt and hate for us?

In the 1983 American Civil Liberties Union handbook *The Rights of Gay People*,[13] a national survey listed sixteen states which had enforceable laws allowing sentences between five and twenty years imprisonment for consenting adults engaging in a homosexual relationship. Almost all of the other states had some form of criminal legislation applied to these consenting adults. To date, only two states have statewide legislation which prohibits discrimination on the basis of sexual orientation: Wisconsin and Massachusetts.

Nationally, the federal government is no better. It constantly abuses gay men and lesbians with its policy of expelling them from the military; this in the face of a recent research report sponsored by the military which concluded that there is no rational basis for continuation of this practice.[14] How is it that we in the gay community have so unquestionably trusted our government's claims about AIDS and HIV, when this government has and continues to express little but ill will towards us. Remember, in 1989 alone, over 61,000 U.S. citizens—more than died in the first decade of AIDS (1979–1988)—are expected to die from cancers of the colon and rectum,[15] and the most we've done as a nation is to embrace oat bran cereal. Remember, over one thousand people die daily from complications related to cigarette smoking, but our government still subsidizes U.S. farmers with price supports to grow tobacco when thousands are homeless and starving on our city streets.[16] How can the gay community believe that this government's motives, which guide national research into AIDS, are for the benefit of a second-class minority the government despises? To trust your health to those who would be your enemy is surely a fatal mistake.

And so I have come full circle to close this afterword from where this book began: more than anything else, ignorance is the cause of AIDS.

References

1. Alfred Fournier, *The Treatment and Prophylaxis of Syphilis*, Rebman Co. (New York: 1907), 301.
2. This figure was obtained from the National AIDS Hotline (1-800-342-2437), which receives monthly updates from the CDC.
3. Joan J. McKenna, "Syphilis: The Legacy of War," *MINERVA: A Quarterly on Women in the Military*, (April 1989).
4. Dr. Stephen S. Caiazza, *AIDS: One Doctor's Personal Struggle* (Dr. Stephen S. Caiazza, Publisher, 1989).
5. Peter H. Duesberg, "Human Immunodeficiency Virus and Acquired Immunodeficiency Syndrome: Correlation but not causation," *Proceedings of the National Academy of Sciences*, vol. 86 (February 1989): 755–764.
6. P.D. Markham, et. al., "Correlation Between Exposure to Human T-Cell Leukemia-Lymphoma Virus-III and the Development of AIDS," *Annals of the New York Academy of Sciences*, vol. 437 (1984): 106–109.
7. William Morris, Editor, *The American Heritage Dictionary of the English Language*, (American Heritage Publishing Co. & Houghton Mifflin Co.: 1973), Abiogenesis defined, 3.
8. P.H. Duesberg, op. cit.; Dr. B.F. Miller and C.B. Keane, R.N., *Encyclopedia and Dictionary of Medicine, Nursing, and Allied Health* (W.B. Saunders Co.: 1978), Koch's postulates defined, 558.
9. A.E. Pitchenik, et. al., "Opportunistic infections and Kaposi's Sarcoma among Haitians: evidence of a new acquired immunodeficiency state," *Annals of Internal Medicine*, vol. 98, no. 3 (March 1983): 282.
10. For an excellent discussion of adaptive radiation refer to Encyclopedia Britanica, volume 18 (1989): 1000–1002.
11. Holmes, Mardh, Sparling, and Wiesner, *Sexually Transmitted Diseases* (McGraw-Hill Book Co.: 1984), 291.
12. R.J. Dattwyler, et. al., "Treatment of Late Lyme Borreliosis—Randomized Comparison of Ceftriaxone and Penicillin," *Lancet*, (5/28/88): 1191–1194; Dr. J.J. Halperin, et. al, "Lyme Disease: Cause of a Treatable Peripheral Neuropathy," *Neurology*, vol. 37 (November 1987): 1700–1706; Dr. R.J. Dattwyler and Dr. Marc Golightly, "Lyme Disease," *Emergency Decisions*, (June 1987): 26–28, 30–32; R.C. Johnson, et. al., "In Vitro and In Vivo Susceptibility of the Lyme Disease Spirochete, Borrelia burgdorferi, to Four Antimicrobial Agents," *Antimicrobial Agents and Chemotherapy*, vol. 31, no. 2 (February, 1987): 164–167.
13. T.B. Stoddard, et. al., *The Rights of Gay People*, (Bantam Books, 1983), 131–166.
14. "Gays Qualify for Military, Study Says," Associated Press, Washington, *Miami Herald*, 10/29/89, 3A; Cliff O'Neill, "Anonymous

Pentagon Bureaucrat Goes Public with In-House Study Calling for End to Anti-Gay Policies," *The Weekly News*, Washington (11/1/89): 3, 16.

15. The Cancer Information Service (1-800-638-6694) of the National Cancer Institute estimates that in 1989 a total of 61,300 deaths will be attributed to colon (53,500 deaths) and rectal (7,800 deaths) cancers.
16. On 11/22/89, the Office of Smoking and Health, which is part of the Centers for Disease Control in Rockville, Maryland, confirmed by phone (301-443-1575) that as of 1985 there are approximately 390,000 deaths per year due to complications related to cigarette smoking.

Appendix A:
Dr. Caiazza's antibiotic protocol for AIDS.

The following protocol of treatment was designed by Dr. Stephen Caiazza of New York City for use by physicians and was being used by Dr. Caiazza in 1988. It is recommended that, in addition to a thorough physical examination, including testing for penicillin allergy and seropositivity to all STD's, and a complete patient history, especially sexual history, patients meet at least one of the following criteria before adoption of this protocol.

Criteria 1—The patient shows definitive signs and/or symptoms of syphilis, and/or is seropositive for syphilis. The MHA-TP and FTA-ABS serum tests are recommended for serodiagnosis of syphilis, as the VRDL and RPR are currently considered unreliable.

Criteria 2—The patient shows clinical signs and/or symptoms which differential diagnosis conclusively attributes to AIDS.

No claims are made as to this protocol's ability to cure AIDS, though there is evidence suggesting its ability to induce symptomatic remission of AIDS for an undetermined period of time.

Part 1—Benzathine Penicillin, 2.4 million units once per week, given intramuscularly for 4 or more weeks. The injections continue until 2 consecutive injections are given which produce no clinical reactions. These reactions include fever, rash, and Jarisch-Herxheimer reaction. Dr. Caiazza's average patient has received these weekly injections for 6 to 8 weeks, though one patient continued for 20 weeks.

Part 2—Doxycycline, 400 mg per day, in 2 divided doses after meals. The 400 mg dosage continues for 3 months. At the beginning of the fourth month, the dosage is reduced to 200 mg per day. This dosage is continued indefinitely. Currently, Dr. Caiazza has not terminated doxycycline therapy on any patients. A termination point for treatment has not been determined, and it is suspected that medication may be needed for 2 years or more.

Not all patients will be able to use the above protocol, due to antibiotic sensitivity. In these cases, there are other antibiotics that may be substituted, where applicable. Please review the side-affects of, and use close supervision with, the administration of any antibiotics.

Appendix B:

Dr. Stephen Caiazza, Miami, 3/13/88

(This transcription was made directly from an audio recording of Dr. Caiazza's speech, with no alterations. The presentation began with an unrecorded introduction of Dr. Caiazza, and his opening greetings to the audience, then continued as follows.)

". . . In fact, since 1982 I really, for all practical purposes, have been doing nothing but AIDS and related diseases. Are the microphones okay? Everything all right? . . . all right.

"I am of the belief, belief shared increasingly by others, that the so-called AIDS virus, HIV, or HTLV-III, pick your own name, is not the cause of this disease. I do believe that it is playing a role, and a very important role. I believe it's an opportunistic infection which further compromises an already compromised immune system, but with very few exceptions, I do not believe by itself it causes this disease come to be known as AIDS.

"Let me give you a little history about how I got started on the AIDS-syphilis connection. Between 1982, when I began practicing, and 1986, I treated my AIDS patients and my ARC patients in very standard, traditional, conservative way [*sic*] that any good doctor would manage these patients. And with the best care I could offer them, with as much time as I possibly could give to these unfortunate people, between 1982 – 1986 I lost somewhere in excess of 200 patients, which I believe, if you do a simple little bit of arithmetic calculation, averages out to approximately one a week. Now a year ago, I began treating all of my AIDS and ARC patients only for syphilis, whether or not I could prove by conventional criteria that these patients had syphilis. And I have been treating them in a very aggressive manner—I'm gonna go into that shortly—for a very long period of time. I am not using any antivirals, and in that year's period of time, I have lost one patient. In a year's work treating AIDS and syphilis I've lost one patient. Between 1982 and 1986 I averaged one death a week.

"The point here that I'm trying to make is that something is going on. I do not pretend to have all of the answers. I may not have any of the answers, but I do have a lot of questions. Something's going on. There is an intimate connection between AIDS and syphilis, and that intimate connection is such that if you eliminate the syphilis, if you aggressively, properly, and adequately treat the syphilis, clinical disease goes away, regardless of whether or not the so-called AIDS virus stays on board.

"Now let's give a little background about syphilis and why it could be the culprit that initially insults the immune system, setting up . . . setting the stage for invasion by HIV. And by the way, let me point out parenthetically that although I'm repeatedly using the word syphilis, we're talking not so much about syphilis per se, we're talking about what we call pathogenic spirochetes. Spirochetes are the general family to which the microbe that causes syphilis belongs. That microbe is called Treponema pallidum. The point here is that there is a whole family of spirochetes which can do the same thing. This in the United States and western Europe is not an important consideration. It is, however, an important consideration if you wish to discuss the [*sic*], and explain the epidemiology of AIDS in Africa and the Caribbean, because in those areas of the world you have other spirochaetally caused diseases: pinta, yaws, relapsing fever, an entity completely different from what we know as syphilis called endemic syphilis. Lyme disease, which we have all heard about, more so in the northeast than here in southern Florida, is also caused by a spirochaete. So we're talking about pathogenic spirochetes. For practical purposes, of course, the most important and the most common pathogenic spirochaete is Treponema pallidum, the bug that causes syphilis. However, I want it pointed out that we're talking not just about syphilis, but about any disease caused by a spirochaete. A spirochaete is a higher form of life. It's a bacterium, not a virus.

"How do we know that spirochetes can indeed impair the immune system? Well, let me point out to you an elegant experiment done by a Dr. Chandler, a veterinarian with the Centers for Disease Control in the mid-sixties. The work was not published until 1976, but nonetheless, if anyone would like to see a copy of this study, I have the original. Dr. Chandler did a very simple but elegant thing. He took four monkeys, higher primates, the next . . . the animal most closely related to the human, took four of them, and put two of them each in a cage: two cages, two monkeys to a cage. He injected one monkey per cage with syphilis, and he went away. He came back forty-four months later. All four monkeys were dead: the ones injected with syphilis and the ones who just shared the cages. They were all dead. They performed autopsies. Guess what they died from? Pneumocystis carinii pneumonia. Now you all know that Pneumocystis carinii pneumonia, otherwise known as PCP, is the pneumonia, the infectious disease, the opportunistic infection, that kills most patients with AIDS. So what Dr. Chandler was doing in the mid-sixties was creating in the laboratory what we have come to know today as AIDS. And those monkeys, just like human beings, would not have died from Pneumocystis carinii pneumonia had their immune systems been normal, yet all four of them died. Thus, we know beyond a shadow of a doubt that spirochetes can be tremendously immunosuppressing. And I point out to you the obvious, that this experiment was done prior to our recognition that retroviruses existed at all, let alone that we had retroviruses called HIV or HTLV-III.

"The other thing that we have to point out about syphilis, is that since roughly 1945—the end of World War II—we have been inadequately treating this disease. We've been using the wrong medicine in the wrong dose for the wrong period of time. What do I mean by that? The Public Health Service, after World War II, when penicillin became readily available to the civilian population, and by that time we had known clearly that penicillin could kill spirochetes quite easily, the Public Health Service recommended for the treatment of syphilis, in non-allergic patients, one or two injections of penicillin, but a particular form of penicillin. It's call benzathine penicillin.

"Now why did they choose benzathine? Because benzathine is very long acting. I can give you an injection of benzathine penicillin today, and I can come back in three weeks and test your blood, son of a gun, I'm still gonna find some penicillin on board. So that's why benzathine was chosen. Benzathine has, unfortunately, a major downside, and that is it does not cross the blood-brain-barrier.

"Now what is the blood-brain-barrier? The blood-brain-barrier, sometimes referred to as the BBB, is that barrier created by nature to protect the central nervous system from the rest of the body. Many things are unable to get across the blood-brain-barrier. Benzathine penicillin, except for very unusual instances, is one of them. Therefore, you have a protected reservoir within the human body that isn't being treated and cannot be treated using conventional medicines. And the man who I believe was most important in demonstrating this lives right here in Miami, a great and fine doctor named J. Lawton Smith. He's is an ophthalmologist, and I believe this work was done in the sixties or the seventies. I have it at home. He has some marvelous photographs of spirochetes in the vitreous humor of the eyeball, which is part of the central nervous system, in quote-unquote adequately treated patients who had syphilis. So we have known for twenty years, certainly ten years, that the central nervous system is a protected reservoir for this bug. Therefore, we have an entire population of people treated for syphilis who in fact were inadequately treated, improperly treated, treated with the wrong medicine. That protected reservoir can be activated at any time one wishes.

"Now, the other thing we have to know about the bug, the microbe that causes syphilis, is that while, if you'll forgive the expression, in a virgin case of syphilis the doubling time is thirty-three hours, as the infection becomes more and more chronic that doubling time expands into the range of months. Why is this important? It's important because the . . . the antibiotic, whatever that antibiotic may happen to be that you are using to kill the bug that causes syphilis, can be effective only if the microbe is actively dividing. Now if we're dealing with chronic tertiary syphilis, and by definition I am, that syphilis has been on board for perhaps years, maybe a decade or longer. The doubling time of that bug may, therefore, be six months, it may be a year. So not only have we been treating with the wrong medicine, we're also treating for an inadequate period of time.

"But now you say, 'Doctor, not everybody has this protected reservoir, the central nervous system in the eyeball, where benzathine penicillin can't get. If I go to my doctor with primary syphilis it hasn't gotten to my brain yet. So what's all of this about?'

"Well, the Russians, and by the way it embarrasses me to say this as an . . . as an American, but the communists have done the best work when it comes to syphilis, unfortunately. Dr. Chinikoff in Moscow, who'd been working prior to his death last year, worked with syphilis for over thirty years, has some elegant electron photo-micrographs, now in my possession, and don't ask how I got them, showing within hours—repeat—within hours of primary syphilitic infection, the spirochaete has screwed itself right into the nervous system, within hours, and we've got the pictures to prove it. This is why, by the way, syphilis doesn't hurt. One of the ways the doctor, in his office, clinically differentiates between syphilis—primary syphilis—and primary herpes which can look identical, is to ask the patient, 'Does that lesion hurt?' And if the patient says, 'Oy, does it hurt!', you can be pretty sure it's herpes. If the patient says, 'No, it doesn't hurt at all,' you can be pretty sure it's syphilis. Why doesn't that lesion hurt? Because the nerve tissues surrounding the lesion have been destroyed by the entrance of the microbe into the nerve tissue. Therefore, if the doctor has enough reason to treat a patient for syphilis, it is my contention that the doctor must go all the way, must bite the entire nine yards, and treat for neurosyphilis. This, by the way, is why I do not subject my patients to lumbar punctures. Because if I'm going to treat for syphilis in any of its stages, it is incumbent upon me to treat for neurosyphilis.

"Now the other element in this equation of tragedy and disaster that we have to discuss are the tests we use to diagnose syphilis with. Because I'm sure you're all thinking out there, 'Well, I've been to my doctor and he's done the test and I don't have syphilis. Yet I have AIDS, or I have ARC, or I have a friend who died or who is dying, and he has been tested for syphilis. He doesn't have it.' Unfortunately, the tests for syphilis, which have never been that good, are worse than they ever were, especially in an HIV positive individual. Don't forget, all the tests we use routinely to diagnose syphilis are based on a normal immune system. They are immunologically based tests. Now, is it so astonishing to think that if you're immune system is impaired, for whatever reason, whether because you had syphilis, whether because you have AIDS, whether because the doctor has impaired your immune system because you're going to get your sister's kidney, whatever the reason you have an impaired immune system, is it so unreasonable to suppose that a test based for its accuracy, its sensitivity, on a functioning immune system, isn't going to work? Not to me.

"The other thing I would point out to you is that which every good textbook of medicine will assure you does not exist, has recently been reported in the medical literature by one of the finest investigators into syphilis going, Dr. Edward Tramont, M.D., who works with the military. As you know, syphilis can be divided into various stages: primary, secondary, tertiary. Secondary syphilis is the syphilis associated with the body rash that we've all heard about. If you read any decent textbook of medicine, any good textbook of infectious diseases you will read that seronegative secondary syphilis does not exist. Let me translate that medical jargon into layman's jargon. Seronegative means no evidence by blood testing. Seronegative secondary syphilis was always thought to be an impossibility. It does not exist . . . all right? Ed Tramont reported three months ago in the *Annals of Internal Medicine* the existence of seronegative secondary syphilis in an HIV positive individual. Now if seronegative secondary syphilis exists, and we've now proven that, why can't seronegative tertiary syphilis exist? Of course it can.

"I suspected that something like this was going on back in 1985. As I mentioned to you, between '82 and roughly '86, I was doing AIDS in a very traditional and very standard manner. And while I was seeing this exponential increase in HIV infection, while I was seeing all of the other sexually transmitted diseases, gonorrhea, amoebiasis, herpes, hepatitis, chlamydia, name one, invent one, I saw them all, I wasn't seeing syphilis. That is, I was seeing one case a year, two cases a year. I didn't understand this. I couldn't understand how I could see every sexually transmitted disease known to man, at the rates you would expect them in the gay population I was dealing with, including HIV, but no syphilis. Shortly thereafter, in 1986, end of 1985, by coincidence, all of this was serendipity, I had three patients with full-blown AIDS who also came in one day with not only obvious syphilis, but seropositive syphilis. I got lucky. I treated those patients for the syphilis, which clearly they had, in a very standard way. While they were being treated for syphilis, their AIDS got better. The mistake I made, however, was to treat them for a limited period of time, because once I stopped treating them for syphilis, the AIDS symptoms came back and they quickly relapsed. That lead me to believe something screwy here: the tests do not work. And now we know that. We have reports in the *New England Journal of Medicine*, we have reports in the *Journal of the American Medical Association*, we have reports in the *Annals of Internal Medicine*, that if you've, especially if you've got an HIV positive individual, the tests for syphilis are terribly unreliable.

"So that is the historical perspective from which I came. Now let me explain to you what I'm doing in my practice, and some of the results that I'm having. We presently have between a hundred and twenty-five and a hundred and fifty individuals. All of them are HIV positive. One hundred percent of them are HIV positive. We are using no antivirals. Except for zinc, we are using no immuno-stimulants. I am treating all of these patients only for syphilis, in a very aggressive way, which I'm going to explain in a minute, and all of them on an ambulatory basis. Now I mentioned that in the past year, out of these hundred and twenty-five, hundred and fifty patients, and by the way I brought with me today data on fifty of these patients, and I've given it out—you can circulate it, you can xerox it, you can duplicate it, you can toss it in the garbage, do with it what you want, but there's data floating around on fifty of these patients . . . okay?—with the exception of the one patient we lost, and, honestly, I expect I'm going to lose a few more—there is a point of no return after all—they're all getting better.

"What do I mean by getting better? I mean specifically that clinically they are improving. They feel better. The thrush, with proper treatment goes away and stays away. The skin lesions of Kaposi's sarcoma, in most of the patients with Kaposi sarcoma, not all, but most of my KS patients the lesions are beginning to fade. The first patient I ever began treating who had KS, doesn't have KS anymore. It's gone, and he is living a normal active life. I have several dozens of patients who used to be on disability, who were unable to work because they had no energy. They couldn't eat. They were losing weight. They are back at work. They are working five days a week. They are working full schedules. They are paying their taxes. They are supporting themselves. The clinical response is dramatic, surprising, startling, and at times not even I believe it.

"Now that's the clinical end of it. What about the laboratory parameters? What about their numbers? The numbers also begin, after a while, to improve. The numbers, however, lag behind the clinical response of the patient.

"Now what regimen am I using? I'm using the following. Visit number one is a thorough physical and history: physical examination and history, specifically a sexual history. And we look very, very hard for any kind of central nervous system involvement, that is, problems with short term memory, difficulty concentrating, irritability, lose of or diminution in libido. We look very hard for central nervous system findings, because they respond beautifully. And then we do a major laboratory workup, and let me just summarize that workup by saying, just to give you an idea of what . . . of how difficult it is to diagnose syphilis without being able to rely on the standard tests, the laboratory costs alone of the initial workup run between four- and five-hundred dollars. And let me quickly point out, that in the state of New York, by law, the doctor cannot have a piece of that action. I say that because some people think, 'Well, of course he's spending four- or five-hundred dollars. He's getting twenty percent of that.' No, by law, the doctor cannot receive a penny of those laboratory fees. It's a direct bill from the laboratory to the patient, or to the patient's insurance. So a baseline workup is extraordinarily expensive: costs between four- and five-hundred dollars.

"Once we've done the workup and we have convinced ourselves that there is need here for treatment, and that's not usually much of a challenge, we begin—assuming the patient is not penicillin allergic, and if there is any suggestion that the patient may be allergic to penicillin, we test them. There's a very easy simple way to find out whether or not any given individual is allergic to penicillin. And I have found in my practice that the incidence of true penicillin allergy, regardless of the history the patient gives you, is remarkably low. I have maybe three or four, five perhaps, truly penicillin allergic patients out of that hundred twenty-five, hundred and fifty. Therefore, we start with weekly injections of penicillin, one injection a week. Well, now what kind of penicillin and how much? I use the benzathine penicillin which I've just so severely criticized. Why I do that, I'll explain in a minute. We use two-point-four million units per injection, which by the way is not an excessive dose. It's the standard dose for the treatment of syphilis recommended by the Centers for Disease Control. From there, however, everything changes and I'm doing everything differently.

"The patient will receive one of these injections per week for X number of weeks. Now what does the X stand for? The X stands for a minimum of four injections. I'm averaging between six and eight, but I have gone as high as twenty. Well, how do I decide how many injections to give? Roughly speaking, eighty percent of the patients whom you give an injection to, regardless of what their blood tells you in terms of their status for syphilis, will have some kind of short-lived reaction. That is, within twelve, eighteen, twenty-four hours of having received the injection, the patient will have a low grade fever, aches and pains, feel like he has the flu. That will last a day. Some of the patients have what we call a full-blown Jarisch-Herxheimer reaction, which is a fever of a hundred and two, a hundred and four, you feel miserable, you think you're gonna die. It lasts twenty-four hours. It's gone like that. I've had several patients who have repeated Jarisch-Herxheimer reactions. By the way, a Jarisch-Herxheimer reaction, the mechanism of which we do not understand, is specific for syphilis. It doesn't happen in any other disease. And in the data that I have passed out, you'll see several patients with a negative history of syphilis, non-reactive serologies, but who had a full-blown Jarisch-Herxheimer. Clearly, they have syphilis.

"Now, when the patient comes in to me and says, 'That injection you gave me last week, nothing happened.' I give one more. And if I can get two injections in a row, or two non-responses in a row, I stop, and I convert the patient to a medicine taken by mouth called doxycycline. Now, doxycycline is a synthetic tetracycline. It is fully absorbed on a full stomach, so you don't have to worry about that problem. You take it only twice a day, so it's convenient. The dose that I'm using is four-hundred milligrams a day, which is a high dose. It's taken after meals. Its side-effects include photosensitivity, loose bowel movements which are very easy to control with acidophilus or a medicine called nystatin—not really a complication, but an inconvenience. Again, it's a medicine that has very little in terms of downside or complications. We keep the doxycycline on board for approximately three months. We then cut, at month four, to two hundred milligrams, and we keep two hundred milligrams going, or medicine once a day, indefinitely.

"I don't know when to stop treating these patients. I have not stopped treating any of these patients. The Russians treat syphilis, I'm told, for two years, and that's without a severely compromised immune system. The entire question of maintenance therapy now raises its unpleasant head. There are some researchers who believe that once you have syphilis, rather like herpes, you have it for life. So maybe maintenance medicine will have to be used. On the other hand, these are good questions, the answers to which I don't know, but they have to be . . . the questions have to be answered.

"Now, let's make a few general points. One of the points I want to make is that barring allergy, and, again, if we're at all suspicious we look for allergy, I can't hurt the patient. Penicillin by injection never hurt anyone, well, except for the pain at the site of injection. All right? Doxycycline, again, unless you're allergic to it, and if you're aware of the photosensitivity that might happen, and the loose bowel movements, and unless you're a pregnant women, okay, but how . . . "

(There is a break in the taping of approximately thirty seconds, during which time the recording tape was changed. Dr. Caiazza's unrecorded statements were concerned with doxycycline being inappropriate to use with pregnant women.)

"There's an expression in medicine, a Latin phrase, and it goes something like 'primum non nocere'. Loosely translated it means 'first, do no harm'. And although I've received a great deal of criticism for what I'm doing, no one, yet, has criticized me for using a medicine that can hurt someone. I want that point taken into account, because unlike other medicines, specifically AZT, some other experimental modalities which do have major downsides, I can't hurt anyone. The patients are getting better. They are feeling well. Their AIDS is going away. Something good is happening.

"Now, of course, the big question is will this remission—and I do not use the word cure, I do not claim to have ever cured anyone, but I do say that I can induce remission, I can induce remission relatively easily, without causing the patient great inconvenience, and quite cheaply. In terms of cost, a reporter and I sat down one . . . one day and we actually tried to figure out how much all of this costs. We added up what a typical patient, barring any kind of major complications, what a typical patient, or his insurance company, would spend with me for one year, including medicines and laboratory fees and all of the above. We calculated that a year's treatment with me costs less than keeping that patient in, than keeping an AIDS patient in the hospital for one day. So in terms of cost benefit, or cost-benefit ratio, there's no argument here.

"Also, let me point out, because I want to get to questions and answers here, let me point out that what I'm doing is entirely ambulatory. I have not hospitalized one patient to do this. I'm not using intravenous therapy. The patient does not have to walk around for a month with a line stuck into him. It's an entirely ambulatory protocol, and I had to come up with an ambulatory protocol, purely for logistical reasons. How do I get five hundred thousand people in the city of New York into the hospital? Figure that one out, inform me and let me know. So we had to come up with an ambulatory regimen.

"Now let me say, what's your job? I mean, what can the patients do? Well, unfortunately, I learned very, very early on that this problem is not gonna be settled from the top down. That is, when I returned from Germany a year and a half ago, I was very excited, I really knew we were on to something, and I thought, 'Wow, the public health officials and my colleagues, the doctors, are gonna welcome me with open arms.' Instead, they welcomed me with a couple of bushels of bricks. Why this is happening, why there's . . . why this issue has become so politicized, I do not know. But it is up to the patients, I like to call 'it patient power,' to educate the doctors. Remember, the medical establishment of which I am a part, and very proud to be a part, is a very conservative, very powerful, very entrenched establishment which changes slowly. Therefore, it is up to the patients to make the doctors realize that syphilis is playing a major role here.

"In conclusion, I want to give you a worst-case scenario for my work. Let's assume that I am wrong when I say that the initial insult to the immune system is some kind of spirochaetal infection. Let's say I am wrong about the role HIV is playing in this disease. What then can we say about the data? What's the worst thing we can say about the data being generated from my practice? That it's all irrelevant and of no consequence? No! The least you can say about the connection between syphilis and AIDS is that syphilis is the single most significant source of reversible morbidity in patients with AIDS. That is the least you can say about the work I've just presented to you. That in and of itself would be a major accomplishment. I firmly believe that the relationship between syphilis and AIDS is far more important than that. But even if I'm wrong on that score, and it's yet to be proven, we have identified the most significant source of reversible morbidity.

"I want to leave you with a final message. Please remember that AIDS or HIV positivity does not have to be a death warrant. You've heard everybody from the Surgeon General to the Commissioner of Health of the state of New York, David Axelrod, say that any HIV-positive patient is doomed. This is not so. This is not true. You're looking at an HIV-positive patient. You're looking at an HIV-positive patient who a year and a half ago had full-blown AIDS. If the current wisdom, if the current dogma is correct, there's absolutely no reason I or approximately fifty percent of my patients are still alive. And not only alive, but alive and thriving.

"Please take this message back to the community. Let us educate ourselves. Let us remember that our fate is in the hands of our . . . of us. We carry our fate around with us in our own hands. We're responsible for our own lives. We're responsible for our own health, and it's up to us to make the difference, because, I'm sorry to tell you, the public health people aren't gonna do it for us. So don't wait. Get on the ball. Educate yourself. Make your own decision, and then act. But do so with the firm conviction, the firm belief, that just because you may be HIV-positive does not mean you're going to die.

"Thank you very much."

(Dr. Caiazza's speech was immediately followed by ninety minutes of questions from the audience, which he answered.)

Appendix C
Biological Warfare Bibliography

Biological Warfare (BW) is an obscure subject for most people. This appendix presents a chronological bibliography of BW books and articles published over the past thirty years, not including those already cited in chapter ten. Your local public library may have some of these. If they do not, your library may be able to obtain them for you by interlibrary loan. Ask you librarian for further information.

BOOKS:

1) C. Piller and K.R. Yamamoto, *Gene Wars: Military Control Over the New Genetic Technologies* (Beech Tree Books: 1988), ISBN: 0-688-07050-7.
2) J. McDermott, *The Killing Winds: The Menace of Biological Warfare* (Arbor House: 1987), ISBN: 0-87795-896-3.
3) D. Long, *Surviving Major Chemical Accidents and Chemical/ Biological Warfare* (Loompanics Unlimited: 1986), ISBN: 0-915179-38-5.
4) S. Seagrave, *Yellow Rain: A Journey Through the Terror of Chemical Warfare* (M. Evans and Co., Inc.: 1981), ISBN: 0-87131-349-9.
5) A.V.W. Thomas and A.J. Thomas, Jr., *Legal Limits on the Use of Chemical and Biological Weapons* (Southern Methodist University Press: 1970), Library of Congress Catalog Card Number: 78-128123.
6) S.M. Hersh, *Chemical and Biological Warfare: America's Hidden Arsenal* (The Bobbs-Merrill Co., Inc.: 1968), Library of Congress Catalogue Card Number: 68-15808.
7) *Nonmilitary Defense: Chemical and Biological Defenses in Perspective*, Number 26 of the Advances in Chemistry Series, The American Chemical Society (July: 1960).
8) T. Rosebury, *Peace or Pestilence: Biological Warfare and How to Avoid It*, (Whittlesey House, a Division of the McGraw-Hill Book Co., Inc.: 1949).

ARTICLES:

Many of these articles are listed in the *The Reader's Guide to Periodical Literature*, which is commonly part of library reference sections. For more articles about BW, refer to the related headings in this guide, including "Biological Warfare," "Chemical Warfare," "Chemical and Biological Weapons," and "Disarmament."

1) J.H. Cushman, Jr., "Russians Explain '79 Anthrax Cases," *New York Times*, vol. 137 (4/14/88): A7.

2) J.H. Cushman, Jr., "Army Rethinks Plan for a Utah Test Site," *New York Times*, vol. 137 (3/28/88): A14.

3) R. Weiss, "Biological Warfare Facility Debated," *Science News*, vol. 133 (2/13/88): 100.

4) C.N., "Army Releases Report on Biowarfare Lab," *Science*, vol. 239 (2/12/88): 722.

5) R. Jannaccio, "The University of Wisconsin Hatches Toxins," *The Progressive*, vol. 51 (Nov. 1987) 20.

6) S. Shulman, "Poisons from the Pentagon," *The Progressive*, vol. 51 (Nov. 1987): 16–19.

7) R.V. Jones and J.M. Lewis, "Churchill's Anthrax Bombs: a Debate," *Bulletin of the Atomic Scientists*, vol. 43 (Nov. 1987): 42–45.

8) M. Satchell, "A Plague of 'Hellish Poison'," *U.S. News and World Report*, vol. 103 (10/26/87): 30–32.

9) R. Rhein, Jr., et. al., "Is the Pentagon Preparing for Biotech Warfare?," *Business Week* (8/10/87): 66–67.

10) R. Boling, "AIDS Warfare," *Omni*, vol. 9 (July, 1987): 97.

11) B.J. Bernstein, "The Birth of the U.S. Biological-Warfare Program," *Scientific American*, vol. 256 (June, 1987): 116–121.

12) S. Shulman, "Biological Research and Military Funding," *Technology Review*, vol. 90 (April 1987): 13–14.

13) "Germ Warfare," *Scientific American*, vol. 256 (April 1987): 62.

14) D.D. Edwards, "Biological Warfare Research Under Fire," *Science News*, vol. 131 (2/28/87): 132.

15) M. Crawford, "DOD Reassess Bioweapons' Risk," *Science*, vol. 235 (2/27/87) 968

16) B.H. Rosenberg, "Updating the Biological Weapons Ban," *Bulletin of the Atomic Scientists*, vol. 43 (Jan.–Feb. 1987): 40–43.

17) B.J. Bernstein, "Churchill's Secret Biological Weapons," *Bulletin of the Atomic Scientists*, vol. 43 (Jan.–Feb. 1987): 46–50.

18) "Review Conference Held on Biological and Toxic Weapons Convention," Department of State Bulletin, vol. 86 (Dec. 1986): 40–47.

19) "Infectious Propaganda," *Time*, vol. 128 (11/17/86): 64.

20) "Secondary Treaty Review Conference Calls for Measures to

Strengthen Biological Weapons Ban," *U.N. Chronicle*, vol. 23 (November 1986): 72–73.

21) D.D., "Soviets Discuss Sverdlovsk," *Science*, vol. 234 (10/10/86): 144.

22) M. Sun, "Dugway Lab Plans Defended by Defense Department," *Science*, vol. 233 (7/11/86): 153.

23) "U.S. Studies of Biological Warfare Defense could have Offensive Results," G.M., *Discover*, vol. 7 (June 1986): 64.

24) A.B. Bass, "One Scientist's Crusade: A Portrait of Matthew Meselson," *Technology Review*, vol. 89)April 1986): 42–54.

25) A.H. Westing, "The Threat of Biological Warfare," *BioScience*, vol. 35 (Nov. 1985): 627–633

26) P. Pringle, "Political Science: How a Rush to Scientific Judgement on Yellow Rain Embarrassed both U.S. Science and the U.S. Government," *The Atlantic Monthly*, vol. 256 (Oct. 1985): 67–81.

27) "Report Details Soviet Noncompliance of CBW Treaties," *Research and Development*, vol. 27 (Sep. 1985): 66, 68.

28) W.F. Allman, "Biological Warfare: Lifting the Quarantine?" *Science*, vol. 6 (July–Aug., 1985): 12.

29) "Army Aerosol Laboratory," *Science News*, vol. 127 (6/29/85): 407.

30) R.J. Smith, "Judge Blocks Biological Warfare Laboratory," *Science*, vol. 228 (6/21/85): 1411.

31) J.A. Miller, "Court Blocks Army Testing Laboratory," *Science News*, vol. 127 (6/8/85): 359.

32) P. McGill, "A Coverup for a Death Camp," *Macleans*, vol. 98, (5/20/85): 32.

33) R.J. Smith, "Court Hears Suit on Biowarfare Laboratory," *Science*, vol. 228 (5/17/85): 827–828.

34) S. Wright, "The Military and the New Biology," *Bulletin of the Atomic Scientists*, vol. 41 (May 1985): 10–16.

35) M.S. Forbes, Jr., "Unpleasant but Necessary," *Forbes*, vol. 135 (4/22/85): 31.

36) J. Perera and A. Thomas, "This Horrible Natural Experiment," *New Scientist*, (4/18/85): 34–36.

37) A. Forer, "The Toxic Alliance: Canada's Role in Chemical and Biological Warfare," *The Canadian Forum*, vol. 65 (April 1985) 6–11.

38) C. Piller, "Test Site for Germ Warfare?," *The Nation*, vol. 240, (3/9/85): 270–273.

39) R.J. Smith, "Army Agrees to New study of Biowarfare Laboratory," *Science*, vol. 227 (2/8/85): 614.

40) "Rifkin vs. Defense Department," *Science News*, vol. 126 (12/22/84): 397.

41) R.J. Smith, "Biowarfare Lab Approved Without Restrictions," Sci-

ence, vol. 226 (12/21/84): 1405.

42) R.J. Smith, "Weinberger Backs Biowarfare Lab," *Science*, vol. 226 (12/14/84): 1296.

43) J. Anderson and D. Van Atta, "Poison and Plague: Russia's Secret Terror Weapons," *Reader's Digest*, vol. 125 (Sep. 1984): 54–58.

44) "The Dark Side of Biotechnology," *Science*, vol. 224 (6/15/84): 1215–1216.

45) "Biotechnology Export Controls," *Science News*, vol. 125 (6/9/84): 360.

46) J.L.F., "Shiga Toxin: No Smoking Gun," *Science*, vol. 223 (2/24/84): 799.

47) "On Recombinant DNA Technology and Biological Warfare" (four commentaries), *Bulletin of the Atomic Scientists*, vol. 40 (Feb. 1984): 59–63.

48) "Cancer Cure or Weapon?," *Science Digest*, vol. 91 (Nov. 1983): 36.

49) S. Wright and R.L. Sinsheimer, "Recombinant DNA and Biological Warfare," *Bulletin of the Atomic Scientists*, vol. 39 (Nov. 1983): 20–27.

50) R.A. Zilinskas, "Anthrax in Sverdlovsk?," *Bulletin of the Atomic Scientists*, vol. 39 (June–July 1983): 24–27.

51) E. Marshall, "A Cloudburst of Yellow Rain Reports," Science, *vol. 218 (12/17/82): 1202–1203.*

52) A. Hiam, "Sending DNA to War," *The Progressive*, vol. 46 (Oct. 1982): 19.

53) "Japan's Biological Weapons: 1930–1945—An Update," *Bulletin of the Atomic Scientists*, vol. 38 (Oct., 1982): 62.

54) D.H. Morrissey, "New Life for 'Forgotten Arsenal'," *The Progressive*, vol. 46 (July 1982): 17–18.

55) J. King, "The Threat of Biological Weapons," *Technology Review*, vol. 85 (May–June, 1982): 10–11.

56) "Japan's 'Logs' of War," *Newsweek*, vol. 99 (4/19/82): 59

57) J. Condon and N. Faber, "An Author Accuses the Japanese of Horrifying Medical Experiments on World War II P.O.W.s," *People Weekly*, vol. 17 (1/11/82): 107–108.

58) L.H. Gelb, "Keeping an Eye on Russia," *New York Times Magazine*, (11/29/81): 31.

59) "Dark Harvest: Scattering 'Seeds of Death'," *Time*, vol. 118 (11/9/81): 55–56.

60) "Sterling Seagrave Stirs a Grim New Debate Over Biochemical Warfare," *People Weekly*, vol. 16 (10/5/81): 43–44, 49–50.

61) N. Wade, "Toxin Warfare Charges may be Premature," *Science*, vol. 214 (10/2/81): 34.

62) Z. Medvedev, "The Great Germ War Scare," *World Press Review*, vol. 27 (Oct. 1980): 61.

63) N. Wade, "Death at Sverdlovsk: A Critical Diagnosis," *Science*, vol. 209 (9/26/80): 1501–1502.
64) L. Garmon, "What Happened at Sverdlovsk?" *Science News*, vol. 118 (8/2/80): 73, 78.
65) R.J. Smith, "Soviet Anthrax Explanation is Debunked," *Science*, vol. 209 (7/18/80): 375.
66) S. Walton, "Germ Warfare' Violation Hard to Pin Down," *Bio-Science*, vol. 30 (July 1980): 485–487.
67) "Anthrax Fever: New Report on Germ Research," *Time*, vol. 115 (6/23/80): 14
68) "Gas Warfare: Russia Steals a March on U.S.," *U.S. News and World Report*, vol. 88 (6/16/80): 37.
69) M. Hopkins, "The Sverdlovsk Incident," *The New Leader*, vol. 63 (6/2/80): 11–12.
70) F. Barnaby, "CBW—An Unresolved Horror," *Bulletin of the Atomic Scientists*, vol. 36 (June 1980): 8–10.
71) "Declaration on Question of Banning Bacteriological Weapons Adopted," *U.N. Chronicle*, vol. 17 (May 1980): 19–20.
72) N. Wade, "BW and Recombinant DNA," *Science*, vol. 208 (4/18/80): 271.
73) C. Holden, "What is Siberian Ulcer doing in Sverdlovsk?," *Science*, vol. 208 (4/4/80): 37.
74) "Soviets Victims of Own Germ Warfare?," *U.S. News and World Report*, vol. 88 (3/31/80): 12.
75) "Big Scare: Infected Meat or Weapon?," *Time*, vol. 115 (3/31/80): 35.
76) J. Nielson, et. al., "A Case of 'Siberian Ulcer'?" *Newsweek*, vol. 95 (3/31/80): 37–38.
77) "U.S. Navy Tested Germ Warfare on San Francisco," *Nature*, vol. 281 (9/27/79): 248.
78) M.B. Callahan and K. Tsipis, "Biological Warfare and Recombinant DNA," *Bulletin of the Atomic Scientists*, vol. 34 (Nov. 1978): 11, 50.
79) "A Pox on Thee," *Saturday Review*, vol. 5 (11/11/78): 12.
80) "DNA Technology Unlikely to Develop Biological Weapons," *BioScience*, vol. 28 (Nov. 1978) 736.
81) N. Wade, "Biological Warfare: Suspicions of Soviet Activity," *Science*, vol. 192 (4/2/76): 38, 40.
82) J.R. Gaines and A. Marro, "The CIA's Show-and-Tell," *Newsweek*, vol. 86 (9/29/75): 42, 45.
83) "Toxin Tocsin," *Time*, vol. 106 (9/22/75): 31.
84) "No One Told Them," *Time*, (7/21/75): 15.
85) "Geneva Protocol of 1925 and Biological Weapons Convention," Department of State Bulletin, vol. 72 (5/5/75): 576–577.

86) J.P.P. Robinson, "The Special Case of Chemical and Biological Weapons," *Bulletin of the Atomic Scientists*, vol. 31 (May 1975): 17–23.
87) A. Wolff, "Delayed Action," *Saturday Review*, vol. 2 (4/19/75): 10.
88) "The Geneva Protocol Accepted," *Scientific American*, vol. 232 (Mar. 1975): 47–48.
89) "Administration Urges Senate Approval of the Geneva Protocol of 1925 and the Biological Weapons Convention of 1972," Department of State Bulletin, vol. 72 (1/20/75): 93–95.
90) D. Shapley, "Impact of Protocol Passage Diluted by Senate Compromise," *Science*, vol. 187 (1/17/75): 149.
91) "ACS Supports the Geneva Protocol," *Chemistry*, (Feb. 1974): 5.
92) D. Shapley, "CBW: Army Chemical Stock Destruction May Cost $1 Billion," *Science*, vol. 182 (11/23/73): 809–810.
93) "Convention on Biological and Toxin Weapons Transmitted to the Senate," Department of State Bulletin, vol. 67 (9/4/72): 253–257.
94) "Convention on Biological and Toxin Weapons Signed by 74 Nations at Washington," Department of State Bulletin, vol. 66 (5/1/72): 615–618.
95) "The Biological Disarmament Convention," *Bulletin of the Atomic Scientists*, vol. 28 (Apr. 1972): 11, 17.
96) J. Goldblat, "Biological Disarmament," *Bulletin of the Atomic Scientists*, vol. 28 (Apr. 1972) 6–10.
97) M. Meselson, "Gas Warfare and the Geneva Protocol of 1925," *Bulletin of the Atomic Scientists*, vol. 28 (Feb. 1972): 33–37.
98) J.S. Bellin, "CBW and Geneva Protocol," *Bulletin of the Atomic Scientists*, vol. 28 (Jan., 1972): 2.
99) F.L., "Ethnic Weapons," *Ramparts Magazine*, vol. 10 (Nov. 1971) 4
100) "Destroying the Germs of War," *Life*, vol. 71 (7/30/71): 38–41.
101) L.C. Johnstone, "Ecocide and the Geneva Protocol," *Foreign Affairs*, vol. 49 (July 1971): 711–720.
102) "United States Welcomes Soviet Move Toward Biological Weapons Ban," Department of State Bulletin, vol. 64 (4/26/71) 549.
103) "Bottling the Satan Bug," *Newsweek*, vol. 77 (4/21/71): 48.
104) R.J. Bazell, "CBW Ban: Nixon Would Exclude Tear Gas and Herbicides," *Science*, vol. 172 (4/16/71): 246–248.
105) A.R. Seith, "The Law and CBW" (Book Review: *Legal Limits on the Use of Chemical and Biological Weapons*, by A.V.W. - Thomas and A.J. Thomas), *Bulletin of the Atomic Scientists*, vol. 27 (Apr. 1971): 42–43.
106) "Department Urges Senate Approval of Geneva Protocol on Poisonous Gases and Biological Warfare," Department of State Bul-

letin, vol. 64 (3/29/71): 455–459.
107) "The Geneva Protocol," *Time*, vol. 97 (3/8/71): 12.
108) "The Horror of Bacteriological and Chemical Weaponry," *UNESCO Courier*, vol. 23 (Nov. 1970): 15–17.
109) "Control of Chemical and Biological Warfare," Department of State Bulletin, vol. 63 (9/21/70): 330–336.
110) "Geneva Protocol on Gases and Bacteriological Warfare Resubmitted to the Senate," Department of State Bulletin, vol. 63 (9/7/70): 273–275.
111) S.Z. Goldhaber, "CBW: Interagency Conflicts Stall Administration Action," *Science*, vol. 169 (7/31/70): 454–456.
112) "Chemical and Biological Methods of Warfare," Department of State Bulletin, vol. 62 (1/26/70): 95–99.
113) M.S. Meselson, "Behind the Nixon Policy or Chemical and Biological Warfare," *Bulletin of the Atomic Scientists*, vol. 26 (Jan. 1970): 23–34.
114) N.C., "Germ Warfare and the Arms Race," *Saturday Review*, vol. 52 (12/13/69): 26.
115) "Bugs Banned," *Christian Century*, vol. 86 (12/10/69): 1570.
116) "Sharp U.S. Limit Now on Any Germ or Gas Warfare," *U.S. News and World Report*, vol. 67 (12/8/69): 7.
117) "The Terrifying Armory the U.S. Scraps—And Keeps," *Newsweek*, vol. 74 (12/8/69): 44.
118) S. Hersh, "Germ Warfare: for Alma Mater, God and Country," *Ramparts Magazine*, vol. 8 (Dec. 1969): 20–28.
119) "Out with CBW," *Science News*, vol. 96 (11/29/69): 495.
120) "The Silent Arsenal," *Saturday Review*, vol. 52 (9/27/69): 14–17, 43.
121) R.D. McCarthy, "Biological Warfare as National Policy," *Vital Speeches of the Day*, vol. 35 (9/1/69): 681–683.
122) W. Zinsser, "Nobody Here but Us Dead Sheep," *Life*, vol. 67 (8/22/69): 42–43.
123) "Gas and Germ Weapons—A Look Inside the Arsenal," *U.S. News and World Report*, vol. 67 (8/18/69): 28–29.
124) "Defense R&D Programs Lopped," *Science News*, vol. 96 (7/19/69): 47–48.
125) "Gaseous and Buggy," *Christian Century*, vol. 86 (7/16/69): 941.
126) B. Nelson, "Arms Control: Demand for Decisions," *Science*, vol. 162 (12/6/68): 1102–1108.
127) D.S. Greenberg, "CBW: Britain Holds Open House at Its Biological Weapons Center," *Science*, vol. 162 (11/15/68): 781–783.
128) "Toward the Doomsday Bug," *Time*, vol. 92 (9/6/68): 92, 94.
129) "Scientists on C and B," *Bulletin of the Atomic Scientists*, vol. 24 (Sep. 1968) 31–32.
130) S.M. Hersh, "The Secret Arsenal," *New York Times Magazine*,

(8/25/68): 26–27, 82–83.
131) J. Walsh, "CBW: British Protests Grow about Porton Center," *Science, vol. 160 (6/21/68): 1318–1322*
132) *"Too Horrible To Use?" Newsweek*, vol. 71 (6/3/68): 58–59.
133) P.M. Boffey, "Detrick Birthday: Dispute Flares over Biological Warfare Center," *Science*, vol. 160 (4/19/68): 285–288.
134) S. Hersh, "Gas and Germ Warfare," *The New Republic*, vol. 157 (7/1/67): 12–14.
135) E. Langer, "Chemical and Biological Weapons: Once Over Lightly on Capitol Hill," *Science*, vol. 156 (5/26/67): 1073, 1075.
136) S.M. Hersh, "Just a Drop Can Kill," *The New Republic*, vol. 156 (5/6/67): 11–15.
137) J.T. Edsall and M. Meselson, "Proliferation of CB Warfare," *Science*, vol. 156 (5/26/67): 1029–1030.
138) J.H. Rothschild, "Chemical and Biological Warfare in South Vietnam," *Science*, vol. 156 (4/14/67): 167–168.
139) "5,000 Scientists vs. CBW," *Science News*, vol. 91 (2/25/67): 185.
140) E. Langer, "Chemical and Biological Warfare (I): The Research Program," *Science*, vol. 155 (1/13/67): 174–179.
141) E. Langer, "Chemical and Biological Warfare (II): The Weapons and the Policies," *Science*, vol. 155 (1/13/67): 299–303.
142) H.A. Jack, "The United Nations and Chemical Warfare," *Christian Century*, vol. 84 (1/11/67): 60–62.
143) "Army Fights Bio-Warfare," *Science News Letter*, vol. 90 (10/8/66): 268.
144) W.S. Beller, "Forthright CBR Policy Urged," *Missiles and Rockets*, vol. 16 (4/19/65): 27–28, 31.
145) B.H. Frisch, "The Peril of Non-Nuclear Weapons," *Science Digest*, vol. 57 (Mar. 1965): 8–13.
146) Dr. C.F. Rassweller, "What's so Terrible about Germ Warfare?," *Saturday Evening Post*, vol. 238 (1/30/65): 12, 16.
147) M. Meselson, Book Review, *Tomorrow's Weapons: Chemical and Biological*, by J.H. Rothschild, *Bulletin of the Atomic Scientists*, vol. 20 (Oct. 1964): 35–36.
148) R.L. Pfaltzgraff, Jr., "Biological and Chemical Weapons," *Current History*, vol. 47 (July 1964): 18–24, 51–52.
149) "Destroyers that Leave no Wounds," *Business Week*, (12/5/64): 106, 109–110.
150) J. Trainor, "DOD Weighs New War Concept," *Missiles and Rockets*, vol. 15 (10/5/64): 14.
151) C.H. Coggins, M.D., U.S.N. Ret., "Is Russia Outstripping Us in Weapons of Mass Destruction?," *Vital Speeches of the Day*, vol. 29 (2/15/63): 263–266
152) "Better than Miltown," *The Nation*, vol. 194 (4/21/62): 342.

153) "Gas, Germs, May Decide Result of Nuclear War," *Science News Letter*, vol. 80 (9/30/61): 224.
154) "Gas-Germ Warfare Defense," *Science News Letter*, vol. 79 (6/17/61): 374.
155) D. Orphan, "The Three Deadly Faces of Modern Warfare," *Today's Health*, vol. 39 (Mar. 1961): 21–23, 74–78.
156) J.G. Hubbell, "Let's Face the Truth About Gas and Germ Weapons," *The Reader's Digest*, vol. 77 (Aug. 1960): 77–82.
157) N. Cousins, "CBR vs. Man," *Saturday Review*, vol. 43 (7/23/60): 9–12, 38–39.
158) B. Glass, "Biological and Chemical Warfare: An International Symposium," *Bulletin of the Atomic Scientists*, vol. 16 (June 1960): 226–227.
159) T. Rosebury, "Some Historical Considerations," *Bulletin of the Atomic Scientists*, vol. 16 (June 1960): 227–236.
160) A.A. Imshenetsky, "Modern Microbiology and the Biological Warfare Menace," *Bulletin of the Atomic Scientists*, vol. 16 (June 1960): 241–242.
161) A. Lwoff, "The Possibility of Selecting Infectious Disease Agents," *Bulletin of the Atomic Scientists*, vol. 16 (June 1960): 243–244.
162) Dr. H.S. Anker, "Viruses and Rickettsiae as BW Agents," *Bulletin of the Atomic Scientists*, vol. 16 (June 1960): 246–247.
163) H. Riehl, "Meteorological Conditions and BW," vol. 16 (June 1960): 253.
164) M.S., "Defense Against CW and BW," *Bulletin of the Atomic Scientists*, vol. 16 (June 1960): 254–256.
165) J. Barden, "Germ-Gas Warfare," *The Nation*, vol. 190 (4/30/60): 383–385.
166) H.C. Allison, "Chemical and Biological Warfare Defenses," *Bulletin of the Atomic Scientists*, vol. 15 (Dec. 1959): 428.
167) "Gas and Germs as Weapons," *The New Republic*, vol. 141 (10/12/59): 5.
168) "On Biological and Chemical Warfare," *Bulletin of the Atomic Scientists*, vol. 15 (Oct. 1959): 337–339.
169) J.S. Bagby, "Witness Against Germ Warfare," *Christian Century*, vol. 76 (9/29/59): 1087.
170) "Russians Work on Germ-Radiological Warfare," *Science News Letter*, vol. 76 (7/4/59): 4.
171) J.H. Rothschild, "Germs and Gas: The Weapons Nobody Dares Talk About," *Harper's Magazine*, vol. 218 (June, 1959): 29–34.

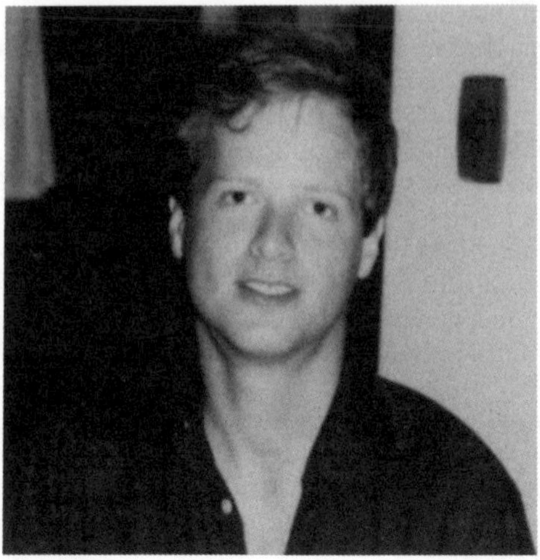

About the Author

Bob Mitchell is currently employed at the Miami-Dade Community College Medical Center Campus, Miami, Florida, where he is in charge of their centralized test banking facility. He holds a B.S. in science education and psychology, and teacher certification in physics, chemistry, and biology. He is a guest lecturer speaking about gay issues at the University of Miami, Miami-Dade Community College, and Barry University (Miami). In his free time, Mr. Mitchell is the volunteer director of the Gay and Lesbian Community Center of Greater Miami and the Gay and Lesbian Community Hotline of Greater Miami (305) 759-3661.

Selected Names Index

Selected Subjects Index

T

U

V

W

Y